LOSE WEIGHT, GAIN MONEY

BY EMILY KATHERINE SCARDINO

LOSE WEIGHT, GAIN MONEY

By Emily Katherine Scardino

For my Drushka, Andrei, for all his love and support, and my family for theirs: also, to my great friends, and to anyone who can benefit from this book.

Registration Number: TXu 1-589-878

ISBN: 1448635527

EAN-13: 9781448635528

PREFACE AND SUMMARY:

This book can be used as a diet plan, but it is actually more of a weight-loss philosophy than anything else. It is based on a concept that helped me lose weight: by eliminating extra, expensive treats that I would eat each day (a gourmet chocolate bar here, a sugar-packed smoothie there), I would save both hundreds of calories a day from going straight to my hips, and hundreds of dollars a month — fattening up my wallet.

I came up with the initial idea to follow this plan back around 2001, and actually finally started doing it in 2006, in the process, writing this book.

The money I saved helped me lose weight, pay off my debt, enjoy a better lifestyle with more travel, and even donate to charity. I hope this book can help other people do the same.

It includes an outline of the plan, reasons to stick with it, some examples, and a planner in the back, so you can keep track of the food you are cutting out, and the money you are saving as a result.

I came up with and followed this concept before the economy started tanking, but based on the current financial state of affairs, it is timely and effective. Based on my personal experience, and simple science, it works.

It is time for my plan to hit the market, to help readers help themselves, and others in the process. If just one person benefits from reading my book, I am happy.

Thank you for reading, and I wish you health, wealth, and success.

4

Lose Weight, Gain Money

How to Fatten Your Wallet While Trimming Your Waistline: Save money and lose weight all at once.

TABLE OF CONTENTS:

6

INTRODUCTION

This is not another diet book. It's the expression of a point of view, and a way of being.

Boiled down to a sentence, here it is: Lose weight and gain money in the process.

It's a plan that can help you drop pounds. It is a common-sense philosophy that helped me lose more than 45 pounds almost effortlessly in less than 12 months, after years and years of struggling with my weight — while finally paying my credit card debt off. I even saved enough money to go on some nice vacations, open a savings account again (finally) and to donate some cash to charity once in a while. I'm thinner, and (relatively, for a writer) richer. And it was the easiest way to lose weight, ever, for me. And it could be for you. My friends, former coworkers, and others have been amazed at my results, asking 'how did you do it?' Well, this is how!

Not to perhaps overstate the case, this plan can also help you save the world, one $.85 vending machine cupcake or

$8 half-pound of gouda at a time. By reducing your food consumption as your weight decreases, and by eating healthier foods, you will both help do your part in helping to stave off an anticipated and perhaps already current global food shortage (more on this later), and help balance out the higher cost of food. You are leaving a smaller carbon footprint by eating less, and eating healthier. You are saving gas (and money on gas) because you weigh less, and your car will get better mileage as a result. You're eating less, using less packaging, washing fewer dishes (and using less water and sending less environmentally detrimental detergent down your drain). It's a win-win scenario, any way you look at it.

I wrote the bulk of this book well before gas prices shot up, and the economy went south, based on my own financial credit crunch and weight-loss issues, but I cannot think of a timelier moment in which to introduce it.

And, my self-proven concept can work with any other sensible health and fitness plan or on its own, just by making some minor alterations — namely, reductions — in your daily diet.

The goal is to provide a new perspective on overeating, to put a positive spin on cutting back (not equaling deprivation), and to serve up information on the kind of foods — and how little of them — you should be putting in your body. Yes, it involves minor cutbacks — but the rewards more than make up for it. There will always be another brownie to buy — after you've lost the weight.

It is also what I hope is an unassailable argument to use whenever you come close to falling off the wagon (or make that, onto the chuck wagon, or into the line at your favorite fast food restaurant). It's a rational, straightforward-as-possible look at various aspects of diet and exercise, and what they mean for you; the big-picture view from 10,000 feet on all of this diet-and-fitness stuff.

Aside from my own successfully tested theory, however, I wanted to write this book because I was frustrated with traditional diet books that were typically one-sided in their approaches. Most preach, sometimes rather maniacally, 'follow this strict, cult-like regimen, because it is the only way to successfully lose weight." But to me at least, life is too short to live under such boring, rigid constraints. I, like you, have things to do, and more important ways to spend my time than carefully weighing out chicken breasts, or keeping NASA-esque logs of every molecule of fat, carbohydrate, and protein I put in my mouth.

Plus, that kind of one-sided end-all, be-all theory that diets are one-size-fits-all standing true simply doesn't seem to be the case. There is a slew of information on diet and exercise, research study after research study, and the fact is, there is little definitive information on the subject. Sure, if you overeat and are inactive, you'll generally pack on some pounds, but beyond that, the theories and opinions start to diverge vastly. It is so confusing out there that I, as I'm sure many of you have, just shut down completely at one point at the thought of how to eat "right" and had just given up, going for what tasted good instead. Some people swear by low-fat eating, others, by low-carbohydrate regimes. Depending on their bodies, personal tastes, and how much they're eating, they could both be right, or wrong.

The USDA has even changed the carbohydrate-heavy food pyramid (make that, food pyramids[1] that had been set in stone for years, recognizing that there isn't a one-size-fits-all approach to a healthy diet (more on this later). To my way of thinking, the only way to determine how much protein, fat and calories worked in my particular case was to see how I felt, if I stayed healthy, if I could perform better at the gym, if I didn't get colds, if I seemed stronger, and I slept well. And of course, weighed less, and lost clothing sizes — i.e., inches –due to fat loss, versus muscle loss. And, multiple pants sizes I lost — from 14 at the max, to a 4-sometimes a 2.

With such wildly varying information, much of 'what to eat?' is very personal, based on one's own body chemistry, to be determined by trial by error, unfortunately.

My goal, as a journalist, is to provide a handy primer or guidebook, if you will, reporting on the various theories and research out there, leaving you, dear reader, to draw your own conclusions. To put together useful information about losing weight — more specifically, shedding unnecessary body fat — and eating healthy, nutrient rich food. The research I cite at various points in the book will possibly, or probably, change in time in some cases — new studies are always emerging that contradict previous old studies. I have just included the ones that appear to back up my own experience, and the ones that have been standing the test of time so far.

The one thing I know from personal experience is that this method worked on me, and helped me get fit. If you follow this very simple plan (that was easy enough for an anti-diet person such as me to follow), you should lose weight, because you will be consuming fewer calories than before, and consuming healthier calories, which should help you feel more satisfied and satiated with what you eat, cutting down (true in my case) on cravings. Eating an entire pound or so of cheese for dinner may taste good, and should, theoretically, take care of your caloric needs for that meal, or, that entire day. But, because it contains a relatively narrow spectrum of nutrients compared to eating a meal with some veggies and whole grains included, it may not satisfy you. And you may not generally feel that well on a primarily cheese-based dietary plan, either. Trust me…I know that from personal experience, too.

I finally succeeded, after a long up-and-down struggle, and you can as well. Not only that, you will likely not be as stressed, you will feel better, save money, and also, reduce the carbon footprint your heavy load is leaving behind on our fair planet. What more could you want from a book — or out of your life, for that matter?

CHAPTER 1: A BASIC FORMULA

First, before we get into the specifics of my lose weight, gain money method, let's look at some overarching aspects of weight loss, and why it can be so difficult to accomplish.

In general, the solution to dropping pounds is elegantly simple: eat less, exercise more. It is basic math — calories in must be exceeded by calories out.

Guess what: yes, it's true, and yes, it actually works. It's not magic, losing weight. This conventional wisdom is unquestionable, based on the scientific principals related to calories in, and calories out. It worked for me, and it will work for you.

But how much less should you eat — and how much, and what type of exercise should you do? When should you eat (large meals twice a day, or small portions five or six times a day?) Is snacking a positive thing that keeps the metabolism humming, or a surefire way to adversely affect your calorie cutting, slipping a few too many calories into the daily amount required to trim down?

These are just some of the confounding factors that make it so very, very difficult to drop weight, which will be explained in more detail later. It may help if you, like I did, use your own body as an experimental testing ground of sorts, and see what works best given your particular make-up, keeping track of your habits and progress.

Again, I am not preaching that there is an end-all, be-all specific solution to fitness and weight loss, aside from the unassailable calories-in-calories out factor. In fact, I am saying the opposite for the most part: I don't believe there is a single diet that's perfect for everyone — there are just too many different body types out there for this to make sense. Anyone who has ever shared a table when eating with family or friends can observe that different people crave different foods — one person's chocolate cake is another man's, or woman's, potato chips. This has been chalked up to metabolic differences, hormonal shifts, and other biological factors, but ultimately, what matters is that people seem to want, process and metabolize different foods differently.

Sweet or salty, spicy or sour, there are certain tastes, and foods, that apparently turn specific eaters on, and lead them to overeat. Sure we are all human, with the same general equipment (stomach, intestines, and so forth) but we are chemical factories filled with an astonishingly vast array of hormones and chemicals, and sometimes medications on top of everything else. This all can impact how each of our digestive and metabolic systems functions.

Clearly, we don't all like the same foods, and our personal tastes can vary by the day, as evidenced by the massive array of foods available in today's market.

Levels of the hormone insulin also affect what we crave, and how we absorb it, rising and falling based on our blood sugar levels. Heavier weights tend to correspond with higher blood levels of insulin, leading to what is known as insulin resistance, which causes the body to store food that is digested and broken down as glucose in the bloodstream as fat, making it difficult or impossible to lose weight. I could cite so many sources here, I simply say, Google it.

If the insulin level in the bloodstream is elevated, as a doctor might tell you, your body will hoard calories rather than burning them. And one unfortunate side effect of extra body fat is that it can increase the level of insulin resistance

— a vicious cycle. I used to wonder how slender people could wolf down bagels for breakfast: it seemed that if I even looked at a bagel I would gain weight. One friend with a waif-like body is somehow able to eat pastries with abandonment without any seeming consequence to her size 0 figure — she's slender, but blessed with a lot of lean muscle mass and a raging metabolism.

But there may be some truth to the seemingly inexplicable, varied effect of the same foods on different people; the thin, specifically, the non-insulin resistant, are not as sensitive to unrefined carbs as the overweight are, apparently, so the impact of the bagel often is different; it is burned, rather than driving up already elevated insulin levels, leaving the heavier eater fatter, yet hungry and unsatisfied, because rather than burning that bagel off, the body just tries to store it as fat. Apparently, genetics also can play a role in insulin resistance according to scientists.

More specifics on this stuff later, and on how substances such as alcohol, which is made up of molecules that mimic the shape of estrogen, and fit into estrogen receptors in the body, is processed differently in men's and women's bodies, which also process calories at different rates depending on muscle mass.

I say that calories are processed differently by different people not as a dietician or a scientist (though, as a science nerd of sorts in high school, I did place seventh in the state of N.J. in a biology competition — yes, I would take tests for fun!), but simply as a professional journalist and studied observer. Incidentally I almost became a scientist, perhaps leading to this safe and healthy experiment on my own body (helped to perform some research on Parkinson's disease at Rutgers University as a freshman, right as I decided I wanted to become a writer.) Many diet book gurus, doctors and dietitians have said as much. And it certainly seems to be true from my personal experience.

I have noticed that I process food differently now that I have lost weight, and that I can eat more carbs than I used to without gaining extra pounds. Though, if I start dipping into the honey pot too much, or the always-seemingly-somewhat-full chocolate cabinet (it somehow ended up going up from the typical drawer to an entire cabinet shelf at some point), I quickly notice the difference in the way my jeans fit…or don't.

CHAPTER 2: WHY ARE WE SO FAT?

There it is; that question of why our collective load keeps becoming heavier. Indeed, why are we so fat? If we keep going at this rate; we might throw the entire Earth off its axis! Why have we been getting consistently fatter as the years have progressed, a trend that looks to continue? There's no question that most of us, particularly those who have chosen to read this book, could stand to lose a few pounds — or more than just a few.

According to the most recent research to date from the Center for Disease Control, more than 40% percent of U.S. adults are obese. Not slightly overweight, with a little chub poking out here or there, but actually obese, which is defined by the National Institutes of Health as being more than 20% above the ideal weight for your height or having a BMI of more than 30, or being about 30 pounds over the ideal weight for one's stature. Not just slightly, ohmigosh-I'm-20-pounds-more-than-when-I-was-18-at-age-46 overweight.

The BMI is a ratio based on weight divided by height that medical experts typically use to determine whether or not a person is overweight, obese, of normal weight or underweight (yes, some people do actually have that problem)[2].

And according to another study, by the year 2030, the majority of U.S. adults could be overweight and obese by 2030[3].

According to the Center for Disease Control, CDC a tremendous, alarming 66.3% of non-institutionalized adults age 20 and over are already overweight or obese right now, with a full 32 percent of this number being obese[4].

We are, pardon the pun, in big trouble.

But again, the question: why are we so fat, as a collective? How did we get to this point? There are many probable reasons that the average weight has skyrocketed over the years.

Reason one? The sheer availability of an amazingly broad array of foodstuffs. We have a very varied diet, and perhaps our appetites are mimicking, according to scientists, a healthy craving for variety in 'the wild' that would prevent possible malnutrition. It is a reason why our taste buds are often in seventh heaven when they experience different flavors. If we only ever wanted to eat one food, we could end up severely deficient in important vitamins. And we wouldn't want to eat it as much. A number of plants have actually evolved to take advantage of this trait — one type of lettuce will be missing a critical amino acid found in another type of plant, forcing bunnies and deer to nibble on them both, using taste as a way to differentiate the plants' flavors. It helped plants survive, driving varied foraging in animals, all based on varied nutrition in the plants.

Studies have shown that rats and sheep eat more when they have a variety of flavors and textures to choose from[5]. One would guess, based on the variety of restaurants out there, and the typical selection of menu items, that the same likely goes for us, one might call it the "smorgasbord" or "buffet" effect. If there are chips and salsa, and guacamole, versus just some plain chips and salsa, on hand, one might make an unscientific guess that those present will dip more, and eat more to indulge their taste buds with the guacamole, than if there were simply salsa at hand. There's a reason most buffets are all you can eat — have you ever been able to resist having multiple entrees, then dessert? Who can resist trying everything? My father's answer, when asked if he would like the apple or pecan pie, at a family gathering, would always be "yes." His mother, my late grandmother, made more than 20 pies for one family fest — almost a pie per person (she was a southern belle from Nashville — pie making skills came with the territory.) My mom, fortunately or not, is a great cook too. Variety makes it hard not to go back for seconds, after trying everything on the menu.

Face it, taste matters; if you have a low-fat turkey salad in your fridge, you may still order pizza, even though you know that the former, healthier option would satisfy your appetite just as well. How many times have you gone to the supermarket and picked out a number of virtuously healthful items like fruits and veggies, only to have them rot in the crisper at the bottom of the fridge while the chocolate chip cookies disappear one day post purchase? I speak from experience — and I hate to waste food. The body just craves the calorie-dense, delicious by design cookies, versus that healthy but comparatively blah broccoli.

There is eating to live, and living to eat, and I have definitely been on both sides of that tough-to-straddle line in between. And scientists have reported that "supertasters," those of us with unusually sensitive and responsive taste buds, tend to eat a wider variety, and perhaps more, than those who don't get the same kick out of the flavors they eat. It's like someone colorblind and someone with a normal range of color vision staring at the same painting; the person with normal vision can see and enjoy the entire range of colors. Eating ends up being a whole lot more fun for supertasters than their counterparts, something that could lead to seeking more gastronomical gratification than necessary on the basis of sheer caloric maintenance[6].

Two: it is way too easy to eat, to obtain and prepare (or not have to prepare, rather) meals. When is the last time you hunted down or gathered up your dinner? There is a countless array of food that is easy to make that takes seconds to zap in the microwave, or is pre-packaged (again, not great for the environment), pre-prepared and ready to eat. The only calories burned in preparation involve the not-so-massive effort of peeling the lid off, and grabbing a fork or spoon out of the silverware drawer (after the strain of opening it, of course). Heck, you can buy pre-chopped fresh or frozen stir-fry vegetables, eliminating any possible calorie burning that could take place by doing the slicing and dicing yourself. Which takes seconds, really. Used to be, if you wanted a cake, you had to make it; of course, now you can just buy one at a bakery or supermarket — minimal effort involved.

Another thing: the microwave has also been alleged in some research to zap the nutrients out of foods, like many other methods that overcook items[7]. And a lack of nutrition is suspected of causing cravings (more information on this to come). All I know is that I lost a lot of weight, in part after eliminating my microwave oven, though it was most likely a result of it being more difficult to prepare food, requiring more energy (i.e., calories burned). Or at the least, requiring me to go to the store to buy some brown rice sushi, rather than sit on my bottom and watch television all evening.

As for reason three we have packed it on as a society, eating had become ingrained in us as a form of entertainment. Sure, it always has been to some extent; I would imagine that even our cave-dwelling ancestors used to enjoy chewing the (wooly mammoth) fat, so to speak, around a crackling fire. Even small, adorable monkeys have been shown to prefer to make sure their simian friends get food as well as themselves, perhaps so they can eat dinner with them[8]. Eating in groups has been a part of cultures for thousands upon thousands of years. But we're not out hunting or farming anymore, for the most part.

And, unfortunately, as a former suburbanite, I can say with authority that it is clear that there is not much else to do in much of the U.S. on a Saturday night except go out to eat, watch a movie (not exactly an active, calorie-searing endeavor), and go home. Eating out was and is a huge entertainment ritual for my family, and it was hard to adjust to cooking and eating at home.

Reason four, and this is a biggie, another reason we can't seem to stop collectively packing it is that on portion "control" is clearly, waaaay out of control. Most of us do not have personal chefs or staff dietitians on hand to help dole out the proper amounts of food, carefully rationed out, at every meal. And even a couple of hundred calories here or there can ruin a diet, bumping you outside the weight loss zone. Some national chain restaurants have started to realize this and come out with "healthy" portions, smaller proportions of certain meals that only weigh in at 400-500 calories, versus the 1000-to-2000 that one might easily consume at a dinner at one of these establishments.

It is as if the menu entrees were originally designed to create the most caloric impact possible per square inch of food for the dollar. Perhaps it's a Depression-era throwback of a marketing tool — the most food for the buck is the best value. Even though it might be the worst, health-wise, for the consumer.

Some eateries, reluctantly, due to legal regulations or public pressure, are posting the nutritional "value" (or illustrating the lack thereof) of their entrees now, a staggering shock to anyone. This is the case in Manhattan as of the moment.

The much-maligned McDonald's may seem bad; just a Double Quarter Pounder with Cheese alone, without the almost requisite fries and a drink, weighs in at 740 calories — almost a day's worth. But there are other fast food — as well as non-fast-food — offenders. That burger is not as bad as a burrito at McDonald's former sister company, the

Mexican-inspired burrito-centric eatery Chipotle, weighing
in at around 1000 cals. per order. Or the 1000 calories a
Subway sandwich can rack up — if one does not go for the
smaller, lower-fat ones that are "Jared approved," by that
eponymous guy in Subway commercials who lost all that
weight eating the chain's sandwiches. I eat there sometimes
— but I am really careful about how much, and what type
of meal I consume (especially when it comes to the
dressing). With proper effort, one can eat fairly healthy
almost anywhere.

Some consumers must surely be in shock, given that some
states including New York now require chain restaurants to
post the calorie counts for food. The indie film 'Supersize
Me" starred Morgan Spurlock who ate himself sick with
huge, fatty portions of fast food, vomiting and getting bad
news on his blood work from his doctor along the way,
perhaps leading big chains (McDonald's to be specific) to
question the gigantic portions they were pushing. And
"Fast Food Nation," a well-reported journalistic triumph,
and a rightful bestseller, showed in-depth aspects of the
industry, including how cattle, with normally lean meat, are
made fat, and sick, being fed food unnatural to their
stomachs — grain versus grass — causing them to be sick

and need antibiotics, which end up on our dinner tables, and in our own stomachs. (And by the way — antibiotic-resistant bacteria, including at least two killer strains of staph infection that are basically untreatable with current drugs — are on the rise, and a leading cause of death in the elderly[9].

National chains offer "healthy" 800 calories smoothies, 900 calorie sandwiches, and 1200 calorie meal combos. You would think that a fruit smoothie at a place like Jamba Juice would be low cal, but only a few menu options are, and everything is packed with sugar. There are meal packs designed for children at the local grocery store, Lunchables, that appear to be innocent, innocuous combinations of good-old-fashioned cheese and crackers, or pizza, actually, stunningly, weigh in at a daily caloric intake-blowing 500-plus calories per box for some varieties (they used to be more like 700-plus in some cases, so credit is due to parent company Oscar Mayer for reducing the calories to more manageable levels), depending on the variety.

I mean we're talking major calories per serving for some of the packaged meal varieties that have been on the market, filled with fatty meats and cheeses and sugary candies or drinks, and who's going to stop kids from eating the whole thing while they're in the lunchroom? I really don't think a 10-year-old is going to tuck away a third of his or her lunch in his locker to cut back on calories. After all, we adults know what we're doing — and we wouldn't.

Also, the typical 99 cent or dollar menu at a fast food restaurant serves hamburgers that seem tiny when compared with the standard fare on the menu. Yet, at McDonald's or Burger King for instance, not to pick on the fast food giants (they are merely omnipresent across the U.S., and world so they give a common point of reference), the cheeseburger on the value menu is actually about the same size as the original version from the Fifties. At 300 calories, it's less than most deli sandwich wraps 400-900, depending on the various stuffings and dressings); today's portions again dwarf what people used to consider a complete lunch.

The major chain family-style sit-down restaurants, at your local mall or strip shopping center, are just as bad or worse; a seemingly healthy chicken or Caesar salad can easily weigh in at 1000 calories. Dressing is pure, calorie-packed fat in many cases: switch to a light vinaigrette, and get it on the side. Want cheese fries at Outback? Plan to share, and not each much else, well, ever — an order weighs in at about 3000 calories. Unless you're planning on running, say, 25 miles home — forget it. At least the beer to go along with them will hopefully help break up some of the fat in your body (alcohol is a powerful solvent).

Lately, some big chains have been reducing their portions, but not necessarily in response to consumer demand for healthier products. It may also simply save them money, now that the cost of food ingredients has been rising.

Let me say that I have liked fast food (and very occasionally still do). I used to like going to the drive-up window at Burger King with my mom and sisters on the way back from ballet class (double bacon cheeseburger, fries and a chocolate milkshake, please, for a growing 3rd grader)... I grew up eating takeout pizza, and am a child of the microwave generation. I have thought of items, when too young to know better, such as Slim Fast and frozen dinners as health foods. In some ways they are, but by shifting toward whole, fresh, foods, with lots of vitamins, protein, and fiber, I have found myself more satisfied than by any quick fix.

There is absolutely nothing wrong with eating just about anything once in awhile. Drink that eggnog during the holidays, have that melted chocolate cake on your anniversary or birthday. There are days, especially on a long road trip, where only the Double Quarter Pounder with Cheese will do. Just try not to do it every day. Eat healthy whole foods 90% of the time — even 80% of the time — (and not too many of them) and you will be fine.

CHAPTER 3: COLLECTIVE DENIAL

We have all gotten a lot bigger, despite seeming evidence to the contrary. Yes, don't be too proud you're a size six at many stores. It is misleading. I know that when I can squeeze, with some moderate effort, into size two long Levi's, at 5'9" tall, that something has changed with the size range.

Yet, the average women's pants size is currently a modern-day size 14, at approximately 5'4" and about 163 pounds — meaning that many people are carrying many extra inches around their bodies[10]. Pants size has a lot to do with body fat percentage, not just scale weight, so this increased girth is disturbing. I used to be an apparel editor, and one of the most popular, best-selling styles in men's pants were ones with a particular feature: hidden expandable waistbands in the sides, than allowed a gentleman to go up about two sizes if need be after a hearty meal, or due to continued, daily denial of the actual, real size. Big and tall clothing guru George Foreman (of the lean and mean grill) included this feature, along with shirts with expandable collars for the thick necked, in his line too[11].

Likewise, we all know that the Lycra spandex in most pairs of women's jeans and pants now makes it easy to go down at least one size, due to the stretch factor and resulting fuzzy logic thereof.

It is time for all of us to face the reality of vanity sizing: our rear ends really are that big! What was a women's size 14 in the 50s era is more like a size 4 or 6 now, due to vanity sizing.

But this brushing-under-the-rug of our larger average waist size is no laughing matter, especially since it has a lot to with health. Namely coming in the form of the waist-to-hip ratio. Medical professionals consider this a significant indicator of health. It is arrived at by dividing the waist measurement by the hip size in inches. (For a calculator, visit www.healthcalculators.org/calculators/waist_hip.asp).

Larger waist sizes, and unfavorable waist-to-hip ratios have been linked to diabetes, heart disease and cancer[12] (not to be alarmist, but you know if you need to lose weight).

And it is not strictly for vanity that you should try to do so — of course, we all like to look decent, if not damn good, but, health is what matters most. In Japan, for instance, they have recently implemented strict requirements regarding waist size allowances for men and women, due to the strong link with long term health risks and larger girths. This national health program — in a country with one of the longest average life spans in the world — is mandating that 33.35 inches or below is healthy for men, 35.4 for women, to cut down on anticipated health costs, for one.[13]

The oversized waists, and larger clothing sizing go back to the oversized portions — and we get started young on our overeating habits and behaviors. Prepackaged meals for kids often range between 700 to 900 calories each, often with more fat than a child — or an adult — is supposed to eat in a day. Kids can go home and prepare their own food — jumbo portions of microwavable mac and cheese, popcorn, the works. Schools have been filled with vending machines in many cases, filled with sugar-packed soft drinks that can add hundreds of calories to the day, while children sit all day in classes, not even having gym class in some cases.

I was not always a great fan of the gym period, not being exactly athletic, and have been known to flinch in defense when either a volleyball or a basketball has flown in my general direction (they were always trying to get me to play both sports, since I am fairly tall). And despite appearing slim and fit as a child, I was always, yes, picked second-to-last or so on teams with a "sorry, we like you, but...we uh...want to win.") But in retrospect, despite the smelly, hairspray-laced locker rooms and depressing flickering lighting, it was good to move around a bit during the long school day.

Some American school systems and principals have reportedly banned sugar, sugary soft drinks, and vending machine "treats" i.e. junk food from campuses, and have reported double digit increases in test scores as a result. The trade off has been in the money that the food and beverage providers gave the schools in exchange for their captive audience of children with appetites for un-parentally-supervised junk food purchases with school lunch money or other pocket change, and there was also reported increases in attention spans and good behavior in the news. Perhaps this is not a coincidence. I for one don't think I could have functioned quite well on a constant sugar high in high school. And there have been moves by schools, especially in health-conscious Cal-i-fornia under the direction of fitness guru Governor Arnold Schwarzenegger to ban sweets and sugary sodas from school grounds[14].

And the hours that students keep can also set them up for a lifetime of difficulty losing weight. In a time where a baseline of fat cells is purportedly established in the body, older children and teens, who by nature are programmed to sleep later than adults in the morning, and stay up later in the evening[15], due to different circadian rhythms and melatonin levels, which control sleepiness and waking, are stressed by this, and by their schoolwork. Stress can lead to elevated adrenaline levels in some cases. If stress creates the release of adrenaline, that chemical breaks down into cortisol in the body — another compound linked to excess abdominal fat. This is true of the grown ups as well. Stress at work can equal a gut, no matter what your gender is. And so can a lack of sleep caused by overwork and long hours, or even sleeping poorly due to being overweight or eating too much[16]

So, you've heard it all before? You've read "Fast Food Nation," watched "Supersize Me" read the health section of *The New York Times* and watched countless news segments on the aforementioned topics? Who hasn't — I mean, there are hundreds of diet books out there, and countless Web sites and blogs devoted to the topic of weight loss. And millions of dollars dedicated to spreading word about the cause and potential solutions, on the parts of both companies and consumers. Well, that's the point. By digesting all of the information in this book, you will be equipped with a simple yet effective weight loss plan. You will be able to see what works for you, and learn how your body responds to cutting out various empty calories like sugary snacks. By presenting a compelling array of theories and facts, I hope to provide at least one convincing argument — you can take your pick — why you should lose weight and get fit, now, not after NEXT New Year's. Every time you start to throw money around buying $5, 900 calorie smoothies and see the scale tick upward, you will pay attention. The plan itself is simple; it's having the follow-through attitude that's the key in making it work for you. Make it a "new you" resolution, not to sound too Deepak Chopra-new-agey-guru here.

CHAPTER 4: WE'RE KILLING OURSELVES WITH TREATS

Heredity aside, and all (what I hope is) witty joking aside, by changing our health habits, we stand to prevent some of the most lethal medical conditions affecting us today: heart disease, diabetes, and many types of cancer.

These illnesses account for the majority of deaths in the U.S. today.

You've heard it many times: Heart disease kills the most men, and women, and more than 80 million men and women in the United States have cardiovascular disease.[17]

Meanwhile, diabetes impacts more than 20 million U.S. citizens, and this number is expected to rise in coming years. Approximately 6.2 million Americans are unaware they have the disease that claims more than 220,000 lives per year, through complications including kidney failure, and a higher likelihood of heart disease[18].

There is a diabetes crisis in the country due to the, well, garbage that people are encouraged to eat, because it's marketed heavily, because it's filled with craving-inducing sugar and corn syrup, a substance with an extremely high glycemic index. Right now, the corn syrup marketers have come out with a campaign saying it's natural and the same as honey or other sweeteners. True, it is natural, but it burns off like fire in the body, with a higher glycemic index than fructose or honey, and can change blood sugar levels rapidly, leading to cravings, and, like other sugars, with their high-low insulin rollercoaster ride, possible overeating.[19]

Diabetes is, of course, a terrible disease. And what is even more terrible is how many people have been developing Type 2 diabetes based on poor eating habits, in particular, eating too much sugar. It can be managed through medication for some people, but has dire, long-term health consequences.

It is life-threatening disease. It can strike anyone, but there are definite links to obesity involved. Which means it's time to drop some weight. Those with a BMI of 25 or greater are considered at risk.[20]

Medical experts say that even a 5 or 10 pound weight loss can have a positive impact on this type of diabetes — sometimes to the point where medication is unnecessary. As stated, one doesn't have to be overweight to have this type of diabetes, but there is an established link.

CHAPTER 5: THE PLAN

So enough background, and buildup: Here is the plan.

Since I was having trouble losing weight for myself, I decided to follow it for me — and someone else. For my family, for my friends, and to — hopefully — help complete strangers.

This is how it started. I think that I was like many people carrying extra weight, who put their own health at risk, eating unhealthy food late in the evening, and staying at work or working at home too late to squeeze in some exercise here and there. I certainly had been guilty of that, plugging away at the computer like a (dexterous) pack mule until 8 or 9 at night, working full days on weekends. This was all for relatively paltry pay, and I was putting my health at risk as a result. I became completely, absolutely, fed up with it.

I was stuck with extra fat on my body and a very slim bank account. Make that, thousands of dollars worth of debt, causing me loads of stress that, in a vicious cycle, contributed to overeating. All my hard work as an editor was only making an impact on one bottom line — the one I could see in bas-relief in the three-way mirror trying on swimsuits. I'm sure that many of you can relate. Not to sound completely vain, but there were a few times I was reduced to tears seeing how I could barely zip pants up, or how I looked in a bikini.

To trim back on excess calories, after I finally hit a breaking point (some more on this in a later chapter) I trimmed back on excess spending. Every day, I pared back on one or two snacks, sodas, gourmet coffees, packages of candy, and the like. It is amazing how fast it all adds up, to a massive savings of both calories and cash.

As mentioned earlier, not only did following this plan allow me to lose weight — more than 45 pounds — more easily than I ever had in my life, it also enabled me to do something else that had been very difficult: to save money. These were both critical objectives in my life. It sounds like a cliché, to have taken control of my life, and (though there is no such thing as control over one's life unfortunately) to a degree, I did.

As an editor living in Manhattan, charity began at home, as in being able to actually afford healthy, good food versus going to press events to have a decent chow down, but I have been able to give more money to various good causes than in the past as well.

That leads to an even more important benefit I reaped from this plan: feeling good about myself. By not being weak and caving in to cravings that gave me a quick fix and made me feel good in the short term, but were very bad for me, I developed a better sense of self-worth, and higher self-esteem. Yes, I do eat the occasional piece of chocolate (which I might stress is allegedly filled with healthful antioxidants). But for the most part, I restrict my spending to food that is healthful. Sweets, extra snacks, are a luxury — and can be a vice.

Continually learning of the thousands of people harmed in natural disasters across the globe each year, due to earthquakes, floods or drought-induced famine — starving to death in some cases — I did not feel as bad, knowing I had cut back on hundreds of dollars worth of "worthless" food, snacks, and candy, and could contribute to a higher cause. Why are we using peanuts to make fattening candy bars, when they could be used to feed the starving, as a calorie-packed foodstuff? We are so lucky we generally do not have to worry about putting food on the table, but we should worry more about what kind, and how much, we are serving up.

So the basic premise of the plan is simple: cut back on spending on unnecessary, nutritionally useless snacks; lose weight, and gain money. And, whenever possible, swap a lower-calorie, lower-priced meal in to replace the fattening fare I had been eating. For instance, having a diet or unsweetened iced tea (zero calories) in lieu of a regular, sweetened or as they say in the south, "sweet" iced tea (300 or so calories of, mainly, sugar).

TRADING DOWN: Another aspect of this plan is food substitution — to save a few bucks, and more than a few calories. Instead of ordering that 500-calorie milkshake, switch to an ice cream soda, or frozen yogurt float for example. You'll still cut back on spending, and trim down, without denying yourself the experience completely — 'cause that's no fun.

This food substitution will also help trick your brain into thinking you've consumed more than you have. Drink a large, unsweetened iced tea with an apple instead of having coffee and coffee cake. It may not taste as good to some of you (well, most of you), but it should make you feel better, and get rid of your hunger pangs. Put some honey or cinnamon on the apple if that makes it tastier, or eat it with some low-fat cheese.

(I found that letting myself get too hungry equaled feeling terrible, and then overeating, typically something terribly unhealthy, or too much of whatever I could get my hands on.)

Another option; make your own healthy smoothie with skim milk or juice, a banana or some blackberries and raspberries, and some protein powder.

The reason I do focus so much on easy-to-prepare, and prepared foods in this book is that most of use are dependent on stopping by eateries for sustenance. I am often just too lazy, or more fairly, tired over tasked with errands, work, commuting, to pack a lunch. And I savor the adventure of figuring out what lunch is going to be, and going out and getting it, versus knowing that a half-day-old sandwich is waiting in the fridge. It is all a matter of knowing what you are paying for across that counter: some quality nutrition, or a ticket to high cholesterol and tight pants.

Life is too short for complete self-denial — there has to be a healthy balance between self-discipline and a bit of hedonism now and then. But, not to do TOO much, too often.

SAMPLE DAY'S DIET

Here's a graphic, at-a-glance "formula" you can use as an example of how to follow my plan, based on what I did:

DAY ONE
BREAKFAST: Made iced coffee (est. 50 cents, 30 calories for skim milk), skipped frozen coffee beverage
ESTIMATED MONEY SAVED (EMS): $5
ESTIMATED CALORIES SAVED (ECS): 600 cal.

LUNCH: low-fat tuna wrap, skipped buying chips
EMS: $1.75 (cost of the chips)

ECS: 200 cal.

SNACK: kept on walking past the vending machine candy, ate an apple from home instead ($0.50)
EMS: $0.85
ECS: 300 cal.

DINNER: cooked at home, chicken and vegetables (cost about $3 per person, saved at least $10 on eating out, and at least 200 calories estimated).
EMS: $10
ECS: 200 cal.

TOTAL DAILY MONETARY SAVINGS/MONEY SAVED (EMS): approximately $17.00
TOTAL ESTIMATED DAILY CALORIC SAVINGS (ECS): about 700 calories

(See the back of this book for a handy planner.)

Let's break it down again:

SAMPLE DIET

BREAKFAST:

ESTIMATED MONEY SAVED (EMS):

ESTIMATED CALORIES SAVED (ECS):

LUNCH:

EMS:

ECS:

SNACK:

EMS:

ECS:

DINNER:

EMS:

ECS:

TOTAL DAILY EMS:

TOTAL DAILY ECS:

Now, take this estimated savings and extrapolate it out through a week, to multiple days, or by the number of people per household. That's a savings of, give or take a few dollars, and a meal or two out on the weekend, at least $10 per day. So, you're talking about a savings of $70-$100 per week per person — easily — through food substitutions, cutting back, and making healthier, more economical food choices. That's a lot of dough! It isn't millions, but it's enough to pay off a credit card, or even just save a few bucks. After all, a dinner at a restaurant can easily add up to more than 1000 calories, with dessert and drinks on top — a lot more than that. And a month of eating out can easily put $500-$1000 on your credit card.

It is less than likely you will overindulge on healthy foods — and even a few squares of a chocolate bar here and there won't hurt with that kind of caloric (and economic) savings. I actually found that a dinner out tasted better (usually at a better restaurant with higher quality food since I was saving money, like a nice sushi joint) when I was started eating healthy most of the week.

You are saving money to easily put away at least $4000 to $5000 in a year alone, conservatively, for a household,

$10,000, or $20,000 and sparing enough calories to lose a healthy and safe couple of pounds of fat a week. Without even working out, though I highly recommend it, for your overall health.

It seems so almost ridiculously simple — and that is the beauty of it. It IS simple! Just cut back one or two extra snacks per day, the ones that are filled with empty calories, and add up how much money you save each day, while losing weight.

You know you aren't doing your body any good by eating, say, a package of gummy bears, or a steak with melted butter on top (or the potato next to it heavily laden with sour cream). They may taste good, but that is simply that unfortunate leftover survival mechanism we have inherited, to crave sweet and calorie-packed foods, especially when hungry, to keep our fat stores up. Cut back because it is good for you, and good for others, and you will not feel deprived. We are used to viewing food, especially sweets or "goodies," as treats, a synonym with rewards. Remind yourself that you are not losing out — you are doing this for yourself, because you deserve to look and feel good — healthy, and good about yourself, improving your self

image, even your love life. There are many other things —
exercise, like taking a nice hike through the woods for one
— that are much more fun. Watch your favorite TV shows
from an elliptical trainer or treadmill to keep your body
occupied — not spending your free time keeping yourself
busy by eating snacks for an hour straight. We are
habituated to watching television shows and movies while
eating the whole time. During movies, I've chewed
sugarless gum to keep my mouth busy, and at home, I have
even turned to knitting to keep my hands busy — and out
of the pantry.

Those snacks and "treats" that surround you are hundreds
of calories that have zero nutritional value, and, aside from
tasting pretty darn good, are a waste of your hard-earned
dollars — and will ruin your waistline in the process.

We have been paying to get fat, and paying the price of
being fat, which can range from anything from poor health,
to low self esteem, to a poor perception by others in
society, even, according to at least one research study, to
lower pay and workplace discrimination. And I am not just
talking about headline-making weight-based discrimination
cases — flight attendants and Las Vegas cocktail waitresses

having size limitations — but general stereotypes that overweight people are lazy or dimwitted (what about Benjamin Franklin defying that cliché?), or unhealthy and will miss a lot of work (this could be true of anyone, of any shape). Oprah, a brilliant and accomplished woman, who has done so much good for people, often makes headlines just because she has gained or lost a few pounds — being praised and maligned, respectively. It is ridiculous. Many magazines would not exist if they did not hang in the balance on the weight of every starlet that ever spent 15 minutes on a reality show. I'm pretty certain that my IQ didn't change when I shifted from slender to overweight back to slender. Though as I used to say in college, my GPA does not correspond to my bra cup size, thank you very much (since that metric had shifted to D+ in that time frame due to some dining hall-induced weight gain).

You can also estimate how many fewer calories you are consuming on a daily basis, in addition to tracking how many dollars you save. I did at points, when I tried to gauge how much I was eating while still being able to lose weight consistently.

I found it far easier to focus on what I didn't eat, or on lower-cost, healthier foods, and to try to maintain the same activity level, including daily actions and fitness endeavors, and watched the pounds steadily roll off.

At some points when doing this diet, I kept more thorough note of what I was eating, from tracking all of the calories I consumed each day as well as those saved, and money saved. When I felt more ambitious, I would also keep score in terms of how much protein and how little fat and few carbohydrates I was eating as well, to try to gauge what my body responded best to. I have also kept logs of how often I worked out.

But, the bottom line that ultimately worked best was to pack as many nutritious calories into my day as possible for the least amount of money, and simply note what I saved in terms of the calories, and my money. It feels fun, kind of like a game, when you are doing it.

So you can also simply track how much money you estimate that you are saving. You will also cut calories in the process as an added side effect.

I thought, why pay for a 400 calorie snack that would leave
my wallet empty, my arteries potentially clogged, and my
diet ruined for the day — after all, as noted, just a few
calories over can blow creating the caloric deficit needed to
lose weight, and it would take about an hour on an elliptical
trainer or cardio machine to burn off the same amount of
calories that could be consumed in an instant with a
misplaced muffin (one that slides down the throat
unexpectedly after that afternoon meeting).

Better to save the calories and dollars for eating out for
something great as a special treat — a night at Nobu, or
Delmonico's for steak — and not waste them on
unmemorable meals on a more frequent basis. I for one
have never been able to follow a strict diet, at least for
more than a week or so. Make that, about a half a week or
so. I hate the word "die"t and the impositions it places on
daily activities and on having a normal social life (ever try
eating a salad when everyone else is having, and savoring,
the pasta special of the night?) And trust me, I have a
deeply committed, loving relationship with food, and could
eat all day. I would love it if there were some magic pill I
could take that would enable me to eat as much as I wanted
without gaining weight. But, even in that unlikely scenario,

I would still feel guilty for wasting food nowadays. It's been a major shift in attitude.

And it hasn't been just a matter of willpower. It has had to do with having a busy, hectic life, the kind of chaotic existence that does not leave room for carb counting or food scales. Who has time to keep track of every single calorie, and fat and fiber grams to boot?

The beauty of this charity plan, my so-called lose weight, gain money philosophy, is that it stays with you wherever you go, and is easy to adhere to everyday once you get into the swing of it. You don't have to make any drastic alterations to your life or habits. Just stop buying extra snacks and eating them! And when you do spend money on food — spend it on food that is an investment in your body.

You can even get cheaper versions of treats you usually like, to avoid weight-loss derailing feelings of deprivation, and still save money and lose weight. For instance, instead of a venti iced Caramel Macchiato at Starbucks at about 330 calories (according to starbucks.com) with 2% milk, at about $5.50, I switched to iced decaf with a shot of sugar-free vanilla or sugar-free caramel syrup, at more like 30 calories, with a similar taste, at a cheaper price (around $3). Even better, I would make a flavored decaf coffee at home and make iced coffee (flavored and not) with virtually no calories (for pennies).

The same could apply to a meal. There are those days when the mac and cheese is calling, and nothing else will do. But, instead of eating the almost 600 (590) calorie large bowl at the chain Au Bon Pain, I switched to the slightly-less-fat-filled 440 calorie medium version. That's a savings of 150 calories a day, which doesn't seem like much. But in a five-day workweek, that will rack up to 750 calories in total — more than an entire plus-sized serving of the same meal (and that might not be the only thing that ends up plus-sized!)

Still, your prototypical mac and cheese is not exactly health food, so I eventually cut back to better alternatives — like sushi made with brown rice, or brown rice with low fat cheese and grilled chicken. Have that mac and cheese once in awhile if you adore eating it (I certainly do), but just not too often.

CHAPTER 6: THE MATH OF WEIGHT LOSS

Sure, you know that trimming back on calories will results in weight loss. But, how much exactly, should you cut back to have an effect on both your budget and your bum? Losing one pound of fat is the equivalent of eliminating 3500 calories per week, according to experts, the equivalent of about two to three entire meals. And cutting out entire meals not only can slow the metabolism, but, make a person, well, a bit moody.

That means one has to eliminate, thorough diet and ideally exercise, an average of approximately 500 extra calories per day to drop actual body fat-related weight (not water weight) and it should be easy to lose at least a pound or maybe even two a week, what health experts typically recommend — not losing weight via a crash diet that makes you lose 5 or more pounds in a week. The latter type of weight loss may seem like a nice, rapid solution, but it is just a temporary change, and if you lose pounds by dropping below your body's caloric needs to maintain its basal metabolism (usually around 1200 calories, depending on height, weight and activity level), then the body will slow down its calorie burning capabilities.

The unpleasant likelihood is that after losing a few pounds of water quickly in a week, you may actually gain fat back in its stead as your metabolism slows down, and you lose some fat-burning muscle that your body consumes when you cut back on calories, especially in the form of protein. Again, there's no quick fix — it's impossible to defy the laws of physics. Matter cannot be created or destroyed according to conservation of mass. And you will conserve quite a bit of mass you-know-where without burning off those calories ingested in some way, or by not ingesting too many of them to begin with.

CHAPTER 7: THE BUTTER ANALOGY

Most of us have heard what I'll call "the butter analogy"
before: "if you just cut out a pat of butter a day for a year,
you'll lose (5, 10, 15) pounds per year" (depending on your
weight)." The same could be said of skipping a chocolate
bar a day, a couple of nights eating out per week — etc.
And in keeping with my plan, you could save tons on
butter, quite the pricey dairy product. Based on your butter-
free life, you could buy a new digital camera to take
pictures of your fat-free self in a bathing suit.

However, the body is a more complex machine than
imaginable — we're not simplistic robots, energy in,
energy out. There's that thing called the metabolism,
controlled by various chemicals in your body and the
thyroid gland that determines whether or not that pizza
burns right off or goes straight to your hips (or gut; name
the offending body part of your choice).

In truth, the body is genius at staying the exact same
weight. Again, this hearkens back to our survival as a
species: if we were to lose weight at the same rate as we
did after eating a hearty meal as we did when starving on a

desert island, we would meet our ends quite quickly in the latter scenario.

 Losing weight means keeping from dipping too low in calories for your body's needs. You can guesstimate this based on calculating your lean body mass and estimated basal metabolic rate, or the minimum you can eat per day just staying still, and then figure out how much more you can eat without porking out, through any number of online calculators, like this one http://www.caloriecontrol.org/calcalcs.html or http://www.scientificpsychic.com/fitness/diet.html), but not eating so much that the excess calories are stored as body fat. It is about creating a deficit of calories that forces your body to dip into its fat stores. (http://www.bmi-calculator.net/bmr-calculator/)

CHAPTER 8: WHAT TO DO

So do what I did, if you take my advice. Simply cut back and save yourself calories, and money.

Slow and steady wins the race. In fact, some readers, used to weighing, measuring, and counting food or calories, may think that this book is TOO simple. It can be a habit we're adapted to; overcomplicating our lives. Having too much stuff, including an excess of food, in our lives.

If so, this plan can be used in conjunction with those more strict regimens that seemingly require advanced math skills to follow. This book can still help you keep track of your progress, and provide more reasons to finally change your ways.

But as someone who has never been able to squeeze following a rigid diet into my life, because I, like you, actually have other things to do, I changed my lifestyle in a more gentle, yet still sweeping, way instead, and reaped positive results. After all of these years of wondering about carbs, fat, and the like, it turned out that the old adages of, "everything in moderation" and changing one's lifestyle do, indeed, actually work.

I was not obese, though I had tipped into that territory at one point years earlier, nor was I in any dire health risk, with normal blood pressure and cholesterol, so I did not need a quick fix or crash diet. But I was significantly overweight and feeling terrible — both physically, and emotionally. And I was tired of struggling with weight as a daily issue weighing on my mind, and my body.

Following this plan made me feel very good about myself, and hopefully it will make you feel even better about yourself — the way you look, and how you are as a person. Instead of depriving myself due to a diet, which only caused me to obsess about snacks incessantly, cutting back on calories actually has a higher purpose. Beyond simply improving my health — I was improving my finances, and others', as a result.

See how much nutrition you can pack into the least amount of dollars spent. Make it a game, versus a chore. Enjoy taking control of what you consume.

I have never lost weight so easily in my life — simply by changing my thinking, and resulting behavior. It has given me a new sense of self-esteem to take control of my eating habits, bringing order to the chaos of a less-than-healthy lifestyle. And, with weight that had gone up and down for years, that sense of control has been enlightening and uplifting — the feeling of working with my body, not punishing it and then having it rebel against me for cutting back drastically on food intake, or spending rigorous hours at the gym.

Creating and following this plan also enabled me to give up some of my remaining vices. For one, I significantly cut back on drinking, something that had become a favored social activity. If you walk around New York City, you will see bars and restaurants on virtually every block, it seems. More than one per block in most residential areas, actually. Manhattan is a place with good weather during two brief periods per year, during the spring and the fall, and not too much outdoorsy stuff to do in between, so social activity revolves, as it does in many places, around eating and drinking. There are only so many times you can visit the museum, catch a concert or take in a show in between. I don't want to, despite my boyfriend helping me activate the extremely helpful accounting program "Quicken" on my computer, go back and calculate how much money I had wasted on food before I came up with my cost- and calorie-cutting philosophy (a trip to Europe? A down payment on an apartment?) Perhaps ignorance is bliss.

In Manhattan, at $15.00 a martini, cutting back on the sauce, well, that's a huge savings for both the wallet and the waistline. If "Sex and the City's" Carrie Bradshaw character really drank all those cosmos, she must truly be metabolically gifted in the calorie-burning department, because there is no way anyone I know with any kind of normal lifestyle in the city was as fit and apparently ripped as Sarah Jessica Parker, the actress who famously played her. And there is no way she could drink like that on her own very limited budget and still afford all those shoes (do you know what they tax freelance writing at?) Better to have one nice glass of red wine, with only around 90 calories given the slender portion typically poured and at about $7-$8 per glass at many dining establishments.

And it was especially tough since, as a reporter, I often went to swanky bars and restaurants for press events, like 21 Club, or the tents at Bryant Park for Fashion Week

where liquor is often flowing — for free — in the evening.
I used to prefer gin and tonics at press functions, till I saw
what an obscene amount of calories that tonic water
contained (hundreds per glass — who could tell — it's not
sweet, after all!) I rubbed shoulders with and interviewed
celebrities.

It is hard to resist a free mojito after a long day, but the
caloric impact is massive. Likewise, the free appetizers and
buffet tables filled with cheeses, meats, desserts, and once,
loads of black caviar. I mean, silver tureens full, at one
posh lingerie event. Or an all-you-could eat buffet at the
posh restaurant Capital, or one of the luxe Cipriani
locations, or a BBQ filled with trays of ribs and mac and
cheese at a clothing event at rough-and-tumble bar Hogs &
Heifers. Or tuna tartare "ice cream cone" like appetizers,
stuffed with sashimi. Or giant mountains of free sushi, and
piles of pastries at a W Hotel function. The desserts… and
the cheese: I saw every fat-filled finger food trend as it hit
New York's party trays — mini hamburgers, rock-like
chunks of Parmigiano-Reggiano, you name it. And I ate
them all, too. I lived like a rock star at times, but without
Mick Jagger's skinny arse or millions.

Plus, business trips are always killers. Everyone is exhausted, typically from flying across the country then working all day — sometimes flying in the same morning to save on a hotel fare. The food is either free at events or can be expensed: it all adds up a gastronomic overdose of mammoth proportions. Some of the heavier people on staff were salespeople, road warriors who lived at restaurants, had hectic flight schedules. There aren't many healthy options at most airports I have been too, and it was more than once I had to grab a bag of Taco Bell as the only food option for cross-country flights back from conferences, leaving from Las Vegas — it was the only option, aside from going hungry for six or more hours, in one section of the airport. I had to eat something, but there wasn't much to choose from, so I turned into a gordita (translation, "little chubby one") after eating a Mexican Pizza here, a chalupa there. I am sure many of you have had to deal with similar food-related issues in the workplace, especially when traveling. Did I mention that chocolate fondue fountain at the Bellagio in Vegas, during a work-related charity event (was that at the Seal concert, Duran Duran concert, or both?) And the pound cake, and strawberries, among other delicious things, to dip in it? Dangerous when one is alone in Vegas on St. Valentine's Day.

Fun, tasty, but after awhile, I needed to come up with a better approach to these feasts. Eat just the high protein, low calorie foods, and have a glass of wine or soda water with a splash of vodka and lime, followed by more plain soda water or similarly light adult beverages. I would limit myself to three of the healthier smaller appetizers (say, a chicken kabob or shrimp cocktail versus a puff pastry-wrapped cheese hors d'oeuvre).

In fact, I guess you could say I was living a "Sex in the City" type lifestyle, with less sex, partially due to moral and self-esteem issues, and without Sarah Jessica Parker's abs…or legs…In fact, I was so busy living the good life that the first episode of the show I saw was when I was in Las Vegas (been there 14 times for work) at a party in the penthouse of the Hard Rock Hotel, where they were playing the series finale, a suite so big it contained a bowling alley. In size 13 stretch jeans from Target…thinking I looked good. Sadly, I kind of did, and was still slimmer than the bulk of the other Vegas visitors. But, still not exactly ready for a *Sports Illustrated* photo shoot for the swimsuit edition.

However I feel it my duty to the sisterhood to point out, as someone who used to work with an art director who did photo retouching on the Victoria's Secret catalog, that all of the photos are heavily airbrushed and otherwise doctored — he was first-hand witness to birthmarks, cellulite (gasp!), stretch marks, and other shocking, unimaginable, not-so-super model flaws. In fact, the alleged reason they don't show the Victoria's Secret runway show live typically is that they digitally airbrush out imperfections that pretty much every woman has. So I hear from sources that shall remain anonymous (I am a journalist, after all, though I don't think that anyone is going to lock me up in jail to get that information out of me).

It's fashion, and it's about a perfect image, an amazing photograph, a fantasy, not reality. Really. And there's a little something called full body makeup, too, which can do wonders over a spray safe faux tan (slimming and imperfection-masking). I was once in the MAC cosmetics store near the Flatiron building, and a self-proclaimed (loud enough for everyone in the store to "accidentally overhear") male stripper came in to buy body makeup to cover up his own stretch marks — no kidding.

I myself, having covered the lingerie market as an editor, have been to events where models, male and female, were strutting around modeling the newest underwear, and the florescent lights tell the true tale. There is nothing that stops you from digging into that basket of muffins and butter in front of you like the sight of some jiggling love handles in front of you!

At least one study has found that people eat less when they are dining in front of a mirror, and I believe it.

And I even worked at THAT company — the one I had ALWAYS wanted to work at, dreamed of working at, the one in "The Devil Wears Prada." I was a shoe editor, in the glam world of Italian footwear (and not-so-glam world of injection mold plastic footwear from China), but ended up eating lunch and dinner at my desk a few too many times before the fabulous cafeteria opened to stay svelte. And that cafeteria was as looks competitive — fashion and figure-wise — as the snobbiest high school cafeteria.

But, back to the food and beverage over consumption, I was also a major caffeine addict before following this plan. Aren't we almost all in our non-stop society, as a chicken-

or-egg Starbucks effect! But, I was also able to cut back and, miraculously, give up "caf" coffee altogether. Seriously — I never thought I could do it. At one point, as I was starting the plan, I was shelling out with the largest sized iced coffee available in the morning, and coming back for a second round, or should I say, dose in the afternoon, mixed in with a couple of diet caffeinated sodas.

That's about a $6 a day coffee habit — $30 a week, $120 a month, more than $2000 per year, virtually wasted! Spent on jittery mood swings, and highs and lows, all to try and keep up with the deadlines, but all the while, adding to my stress, and causing my energy levels to crash eventually, leading to a cycle of overeating and caffeine abuse.

Even when I started to save money, I was hitting the free coffee machine at work for all it was worth. But I found that drinking coffee would lead to cravings for snacks to go with it.

Now, there are some studies that indicate that caffeine may have some positive health benefits, perhaps preventing Type II diabetes, or even Parkinson's Disease according to at least one prominent study[21]. However, between the mood swings and the shaky hands, it was time to cut it out for the most part.

I lost a full 12 pounds after stopping the caffeine cycle (rollercoaster, more like it), weight that seemed to melt off once I stopped drinking a ton of it. And, I noticed I was less hungry. Turns out that caffeine can have an adverse affect on blood sugar levels, according to a Duke University study on people with type 2 diabetes; having coffee caused their blood glucose levels to rise throughout the day[22], creating hunger pangs and making it difficult to lose weight while the blood sugar is elevated.

Like the taste of coffee like me? Have some decaf instead, then. But remember that it does contain some juice, even though most of the caffeine is taken out, so beware of large doses of decaf. A little isn't terrible, but, break the habit!

Other studies have shown that coffee may inhibit type two diabetes symptoms[23]. As I said earlier; these are all theories, and there are few facts to adhere to.

I can now partake of caffeine occasionally (and, some research backs the premise that it can help boost concentration upon consumption with occasional use), without needing a massive jolt of java to start the day. It comes in hand when, say, editing a book! But, I like it in the form of green tea, a substance linked with a number of health benefits, and known to have high levels of antioxidants called polyphenols, which are said to have the potential to help protect against cell oxidation, which could lead to damage and possibly even cancer[24].

In adapting to my plan, I also changed the way I thought of food. I am a foodie of sorts, a gourmet, and New York is a cornucopia of a broad variety of amazing restaurants and foodstuffs. I can't even watch shows on the Food Network without running to the fridge for a snack. Anything from steak to cupcake to noodle shops to fried chocolate bars is there to whet the appetite, not to mention, every sort of restaurant/bar of the drinking-establishment variety that you can imagine.

With eateries open at all hours of the day, from bagels in the AM to blintzes late at night, living in the city and trying to diet is like putting a chimp in the middle of a banana grove. There is no escape: in addition to all of the places to eat and various watering holes, there are also scores of markets carrying gourmet specialty foods from around the world — hard to resist! One of my favorite potential vices was the $99 mammoth-sized jar of Nutella I saw at the Chelsea Market in Manhattan a few years back. That would pretty much undo me.

But, after waking up feeling bloated and gaining back a few hard-lost pounds over each weekend after eating and drinking with abandon, after working hard each week to keep it off by eating relatively healthier and hitting the gym, I decided to change my point of view, and my actions.

Though eating tasty food is essential, I believe, to a sense of well being, without overdoing it and eating just for the sake of taste alone, I started to think of foodstuffs as fuel to make my body perform its best — rather than indulging every sugar craving I had. Just because eating cookies feels good at the moment doesn't mean it is good for you. We are, as noted, seemingly designed to eat high-calorie food for survival when it is presented, because if we were, say, living in the wild in the woods, it would help us store fat and keep going, but, eating half a batch of cookies (one of those foods that seems designed to be as calorically dense as possible — with as many calories per square inch as possible — more than anyone would find in food in "the wild") serves no healthy purpose for modern humans. If you have ever been hiking in the cold, you have likely experienced the kind of appetite that makes you crave half a pan of brownies, and then some.

This "diet" plan is a way to use your higher thinking powers to help wean the ancient part of your brain off of the extra food.

You can do the same exact thing I did, and simply cut back on a snack or two a day, and watch as the dollars add up and the pounds fall off. Or, you can follow any additional diet or health plan you choose — whatever works for you.

Yes, you have to make the decision, like I did, that you really want to lose weight, for yourself, and for other people as well if you'd like. Because nobody is going to stand there, unless you have budget for his or her salary, and tell you what to eat and when to eat it — it is up to you to pay attention to what you put in your mouth, and see how your body reacts.

As noted earlier, most of us know what foods (aside from
the obvious cheesecake and so forth) make us gain or lose
weight (though in general, veggies and grilled chicken will
do the trick) — and there's no one-size-fits all approach. It
seems that just the foods that we crave are the ones that
make us gain weight the most. Maybe because we eat a lot
of them cause we like them the most, aside from any
metabolic mumbo jumbo.

Some of us are sensitive to carbs, perhaps because we are
insulin resistant. For those, diets such as the South Beach
Diet, or Atkins could help do the trick.
Others seem to trim down on a low-fat diet, more along the
lines of the Pritikin diet. There are theories that some
people are fast oxidizers, and some are slow oxidizers,
varying the speed with which they burn off food. There's a
bit more on the various types of diets later, with some
highlights of the popular, and non-crazy sounding ones (by
my humble and subjective opinion). There are healthy
seeming diets, and plain old fad diets. And there is no way I
would think it at all pleasant to subject one's self to
drinking large quantities of various herbs and liquids —
and many hours seated on the "white throne — to drop
some water weight for a week. Don't think "I've got to

look good for the reunion/wedding/graduation" — think long term.

Like I did, please take an honest look at yourself, from fore and aft, in the full-length mirror. Reflect on your eating patterns and the consequences thereof. If eating steak is what makes your pants buttons pop off, cut back on red meat. If chocolate chip and sugar cookies can send you from a size 10 to a 12 in a matter of a few days of indulging over the holidays, cease and desist eating them.

At least, stop consuming half a batch and licking the bowl: portion control is also important. If you are overeating the foods that you crave, it may be better to avoid them altogether if you can't control your eating. I have been there, and while deprivation isn't ideal, it is really hard for me, at least, to just eat one square of a chocolate bar or one cookie! My must-avoid list of foods I cannot stop eating if they are lurking in my cupboards and fridge are the aforementioned Nutella, crackers, and any kind of cheese.

You probably already know what foods you crave, and that you tend to overeat. So make sure you eat up before you go to the supermarket, so you aren't hungry, and you can resist buying the foods that make you go overboard. As my mother always says: "never go food shopping hungry." That's when the naughty things get purchased (and eaten at the same time as your groceries are rung up at the register).

If you can't keep yourself from stopping by the candy store and buying a $6.00 bag of sweets after work because you're exhausted (guilty!), take a look in the mirror and ask yourself if you're doing yourself any favors. If you do not have a clear sense of what your body runs best on, I recommend that you visit a nutritionist, or even visit an online diet site, such as ediets, that helps to tailor plans to individuals' metabolic types and fitness levels. Still, if you just stick to this plan, cutting back on unhealthy and expensive food, you should see results.

See how much you save in terms of both empty calories and how full your wallet is getting per week, per month, per year. You'll be shocked.

Think about it. If you buy a fat-and-sugar packed whipped coffee drink every morning on the way to work, you are not only consuming about 400 or 500 extra, empty calories per day-an amount that would require an hour-plus, actually, more like two hours at the rate people generally go, on a treadmill to burn it off. You are also spending, say $4.00 a day on that drink. Multiplied by five workdays, that's $20 a week. Per month, that comes to $80. Per year, that's $960 a year — on stuff that's making you fat, and possibly, shortening your lifespan.

And that is a conservative estimate of how much you can save. It's a snowball effect, and your pantry will get less full, your bank account more so.

Why invest your funds poorly — and in a bet against yourself? Nobody can afford that. Put your money in healthy food, not potentially dangerous trans fats and blood sugar-spiking sugars. Put cash toward your long-term health, and help bank against rising health care costs that you will have to pay if you come down with a chronic condition related to weight gain, like diabetes, or heart disease.

Think about how much money you will have to pay out of pocket, even with (increasingly rare) good health insurance benefits, on doctor's visits, blood tests, medication, and various medical supplies to care for your (disease). Even with a health plan, having to be on pills for a condition can really set you back.

Or, if you already have Type II diabetes, or clogged arteries, think how much money you will save if you can help reverse these conditions through diet, not expensive drugs — and yes, it is possible.

With each seemingly innocent bite of fettuccini alfredo, or cake, you may be effectively, not to be melodramatic, tapping a nail into your coffin. Except when consumed with the greatest of moderation (but, it sure is hard to just eat one bite of cake: the biology of taste seems to trump cerebral efforts toward self control).

Why would you do that to yourself? This is not a judgment on my part, and I understand — I have been significantly overweight, and know exactly how hard it is to lose weight once it's gained, and how hungry you can be, how much you can crave foods, when your insulin levels are out of whack from being overweight. But it can be done, it needs to be done — and you can do it. It may take time, and it may not be easy, but it is worth it. You are worth it. I finally believed that I was worth it. Despite all the stresses (and there were some serious troubles I had to cope with), I survived, and now, feel like I am finally thriving, and really living.

Your savings may or may not seem like a lot of money at first — but keep adding it up from there. The 80-cent mid-afternoon soda from the vending machine seems cheap enough — but every workday alone, that's $192 a year. I was happy to have it. And, I think that you will be, too. It will at least cover a few cell phone bills.

The savings just keeps adding up. You could save for new car, a vacation, and the charity of your choosing. You can have a flat screen TV (I upgraded from my TV/VCR combo to a 46" and Blu-Ray player) and flat abs, all from following the same discipline. It made me feel better about myself, more secure in both my appearance and my health, and more stable regarding my financial future.

And given the current state of the economy, most of us could stand to save versus spend. It is ridiculously, exorbitantly expensive out there. Many of us spend half of what we make on rent or mortgages or other major expenses, and then buy low-quality food, seemingly to save a buck today, and eat it, then eat too much of it because it is not satisfying nutritionally, and it tastes good and provides temporary stress relief.

You can save the money for yourself — or you can save it for your charity of choice. Or, do both. I was shocked to actually be able to save money, and pay off my credit card. And, to donate some to charity as well. Hopefully, even more going forward if you all like my book!

See how much you save each week, month and year. Perhaps instead of a year's worth of lattes at 1000 calories a week, times 52 weeks a year, which would translate to quite a few pounds, about 15 in a year just from the lattes depending on your current size and metabolism, you can look great in your bathing suit on a vacation to Miami — or Tahiti.

A trip that you paid for, versus shelling out for all of those pints of ice cream and bottles of soda. And, with money left over for the new bathing suit, and the delicious food your body both craves and thrives on, like fresh seafood or lean steak and vegetables.

IT'S REALLY THAT SIMPLE. This is the anti-diet "diet" book, after all. And I am living, breathing, size two Calvin Klein strapless dress proof that it works (at 5'9", as said.) So the dress has a touch of stretch to it, but still, we're talking about a size 2, not the size 12 I was once happy to fit into. I have lost about 10 inches in total off of my bust and hips — each — a dramatic decrease. I wear a size 2 or 4 dress with ease now.

It took a while to get here (supposed to be the healthy way to go about it) and I wish I hadn't taken so long to come up with this plan, and longer to follow it and get the results it has given me. I could not have lost the weight otherwise, without eating less to save more.

There has been a lot said in "self-help land" about changing one's thinking and behavior, but not a lot of options in terms of how to make that happen. It has been black or white, all or nothing, either being on a diet, or way off of a diet, counting each calorie, or throwing caution to the wind.

And the less you weigh (within healthy parameters, of course), the less you will spend as well. It takes fewer calories to feed and satisfy someone who is 120 pounds than somebody who weighs in at 200. I spend far less on food now, and am just as satisfied.

Just remember; this book is not meant to make you lose five pants sizes in 10 days, or have instant six-pack abs. It is a realistic way to keep losing weight, real fat weight, not water weight (the only way someone can actually lose 10 pounds in a week), over time, and ideally, improve your overall eating patterns, health and lifestyle, being fit enough to do the things you've always wanted to, and to actually, fully, live your life.

I have done things again since shedding pounds that I long enjoyed before gaining weight that I was afraid or self-conscious to do, like buying (with the money I saved) and riding my shiny new bicycle over 20 miles some days (a bike I was afraid to get when overweight; I was actually afraid of falling, and sadly, self-conscious my rear would look like a wide load from behind). I feel sad that I wasn't fully living for a few years, without the energy to bike, run or hike as much as I wanted to. And I don't want you to waste time like I did.

Even though I tried to stay fit, it creates a lot of extra effort hauling 40-50 extra pounds around, and a lot of hunger to go with it. I used to work out more than I do now, lifting weights, and was so ravenous that I would undo all my hard work by eating too much, before I started this plan.

It was not exactly the Ironman Triathlon, but it was exciting to be able to bike to New York's Montauk Point, on the south fork of Long Island, and back to a local campground, Hither Hills, and climb the Montauk lighthouse in between legs, without losing my breath or even feeling sore. It really breaks my heart to see people on the streets of Manhattan, in Disneyworld, all over, frankly, riding on scooters because they are simply too unfit, in some cases, to walk for extended periods of time. They may not have any underlying medical condition — yet — but they are scooting from restaurant to restaurant without burning off the food by walking in between. Not because of a disability in some cases, simply because they are so out of shape that it is too much effort to stand and walk around.

They may think they are taking the easy way out, by scooting along and "driving" everywhere, perhaps due to knees aching from excess weight that is stressing them, but, it could just lead to obesity and disability — not to mention, the impact on the environment for charging those little scooters up. Do you really want to live like you're 80 when you're 40? If you do — and let obesity take its toll on your health — you might not make it to 80. You have to make an effort to get, and stay in shape.

Are you going to be healthier than your grandparents? Some Harvard School of Public Health and University of Washington research indicates, maybe not: the average lifespan for obese individuals that have heart disease and diabetes have a shorter life ahead of them, the first time it has fallen since the 1960s to 2000[25].

So please, do not wait any longer. Do not struggle any longer, like I did for years, when despite my best efforts, my weight surged up and down with little stability.

Cut back, save money, lose weight, and feel better.

CHAPTER 9: THE REST OF THE BOOK

Yes, that's it! That's the plan. Track what you eat each day, or just, even more easily, what you DON'T eat, each day, to make life even simpler, and watch how the estimated calories — and savings — add up!

If you eat less, and healthier, you will lose weight — it's a scientific fact. Easily save $5.00-$7 a day by cutting out the snacks and buying a lighter lunch, and you'll save close to $2,000 a year, an amount that is nothing to sniff at. You can save much more than this (again, $10,000, $20,000 per household, more if you factor in all the gas money saved by not going out to eat as much, your lighter load in the car), if you trim back even more.

Few savings accounts will bring you this kind of return on what the average person can put into them, especially given the poor prognosis for the long-term health of the economy. Any good chief executive or operating officer knows to look at curbing expenses to improve the financial position of a company is a top priority when sales are down.

But aside from all the pondering of the current distressed economy and the reasons you should lose weight, this plan is not supposed to be a textbook about, say, performing brain surgery, it's a simple, hopefully elegant, timeless solution to your weight loss problems, as it was to my own challenge.

The point of the rest of this book, in addition to serving as a planner to help you meet your specific goals (see the final section), is to pose various arguments that you can use to convince yourself to follow it, and to finally lose weight. Using a simple planner worked for me, with this extremely easy-to-follow-and-stick-to plan. In fact, recent research indicates that men and women who keep food diaries lost twice as much weight in six months as those who did not, something I found out first hand.[26]

At the end of this book, there is a handy dandy planner, like the one I used, where you can track your goals over the next three months, six months, however long it takes to reach your weight loss (and savings) goal. Most experts say 8-10 pounds on average per month is the max one should try to shed to maintain optimum health (losing weight too fast has been linked with gall bladder problems and sagging skin, and being really darn hungry and irritable).

These are reasons I came back to again and again, when that $5 chocolate bar beckoned, to why I should stick with the plan, and shed the weight once and for all. It was always those extras that got me, the shopping cart at the grocery store filled with well-intentioned veggies, lowfat cheese and lean chicken breasts. It was always that one or two items — the ice cream, the chips, the crackers, that were the easiest to grab and eat when I was tired, and sabotaged any attempts at healthful eating and weight loss by adding an unhealthy overlay of useless calories to each day. And, that were an added expense that did nothing but hurt me.

When you hopefully do take the step to drop body fat and get fit, you can keep track of your goals as closely or loosely as you would like, as long as you are getting results. I know that after about three days of calculating every single calorie I eat, it gets a bit tedious. The least-boring, most time-efficient way I found to keep track was to simply indicate what I did NOT eat (that package of candy from the vending machine, the pint of ice cream I was tempted to buy at the deli). And estimated the calories saved, and dollars kept, in each instance.

Remember; that 200-300-500 calories may not seem like a lot shaved off a single day, but they can make the difference between gaining, maintaining or losing weight that week. I found it easier to get to the 500 calorie deficit by exercising as well as trimming down on food, because I do like to eat!

Think of weight loss as a gradual wedge, slowing trimming off calories as you continue to lose weight, continuing to taper the amount of calories, based on the aforementioned metabolic rate and activity level, that you consumer each day. Because you will not need as many calories if you weigh less. A fairly active 5'6" 175 pound man may be able to lose weight will still eating 1800 calories per day, while a 5'1" 125 pound woman may have to go down to 1200 cals per day to shed excess chunkiness. If someone cannot shed weight on a 1200 calorie a day diet, it is time to check in with the doctor (a good idea anyway before starting any health plan) because there might be another issue, such as low thyroid, at play.

This gradual overall calorie reduction had tripped me up in the past, and can be a sticking point for those trying to cut down on food and keep losing weight. Remember: the less you weigh, give or take some muscle mass, and your activity level, the less you can eat. Generally, it is a lot of fuzzy math to try and compute how many calories less you can eat each week. Even taking the stairs a few days a week, going shopping after work, could add up to a substantial number of extra calories burned, the same way cutting back slightly on food can contribute to slow, long-term weight loss. Yes, it's common sense, but it's true. As you get closer and closer to the ideal weight for your body, the weight loss will slow as well, so it will become more important to observe what you are eating and doing than ever to fine-tune the grand finale of weight loss — and maintenance.

CHAPTER 1O: OVERWEIGHT AND LIFE SPAN

Still not convinced it's time to slim down? Here are some more reasons to drop the extra pounds, if extra validation is needed.

One key reason: possibly living longer — and having a better quality of life while alive.

As far as anyone knows, we only live once, and have one body apiece. Until modern science, cloning, cryogenic freezing capabilities a la Austin Powers, etc. actually become reality, this IS the reality. This is it.

It is absolutely a right and responsibility to make your body a priority in terms of food, and caretaking. Whether you are more of a Ferrari, a Honda, a Ford or a Hummer, so to speak, you keep the body maintained, store it in the garage, wash it regularly, and make sure you use the right fuel to keep the engine humming.

No matter what your other responsibilities are, the better shape you are in, physically and mentally, the more you can accomplish. And for those of you used to putting other people first, the more you take care of yourself, the more you can do for the people around you. Repeat this until you believe it.

I know this from personal experience. I would constantly put school, then work, first above my own needs. I used to think it was self-centered, selfish, to care so much about my weight and appearance, to spend so much time and money on my body. But, I realized that the old adage that you can't take care of others if you don't take care of yourself first is very true, based on empirical experience.

After having the heartbreaking experience of having three close relatives die within a five-year time frame, including seeing my grandfather undergo multiple amputations, suffer, and pass away from diabetes and heart disease, you realize that life is short, and it is your responsibility to try and stay healthy and fight as long as possible. Eating too much sugar is not worth the risk of developing a devastating disease, and there is no reason for it, with the knowledge that we have about diet today. It seems like an uphill battle at 45, 55, or 66 pounds overweight — never mind more than that — but, it is worth the struggle, because it's all downhill from where you are right now, if

you don't do anything about it, not to be a complete
pessimist about it. Use it or you really may lose it — your
ability to do the things you like, your limbs, your life.

Now you know your mileage goes down when your car is
overloaded, and that it creates wear and tear on the engine
and breaks — when filled with luggage or groceries, for
instance. Pick up just 15 or 20 pounds in free weights at the
gym if you are in shape to do so, and walk around a bit.
Now think about carrying around that much in fat — or 50,
60, even 80 pounds. It has to slow you down, right?
Imagine getting everywhere faster, on less, more efficient
fuel. Being lighter, stronger, less hungry, while doing it.

Would you buy diesel fuel for a vehicle that takes
unleaded? Don't mess up your own engine, so to speak,
with useless, "empty" calories. Don't carry around extra,
well, junk in your trunk.

If you can only eat 1400 calories per day to keep losing
weight, for example, eating an 800-calorie melted
chocolate cake for desert will drastically limit the other
foods you can consume per day, as well as the vitamins you
would take in from eating those healthy foods. No, taking a

multi-vitamin with dessert does not count. Get the cake and have two bites, share it with friends, but do not blow the day, and your health, on some ice cream or a pastry!

In fact, some nutritional experts say that cravings can be induced by a lack of proper nutrition, which seems logical. Without enough B vitamins, for instance, that help produce energy in the body through metabolic activity, a person might crave sugar instead for a quick energy fix.

And, think of vitamins as oil, to keep the gears moving. Key vitamins include:
ACE: A and E are fat-soluble, so limit intake, but C is water-soluble, so more is permitted, in reasonable doses.

I recommend taking a daily multivitamin of your choice, men's or women's specific ideally, be it from a drugstore or a health food store. The health food stores ones are pricier, but you can get good deals online from reputable stores, and the quality of the ingredients is definitely better. If you don't feel like paying $45 for a bottle of vitamins, then it is better to take a discount-store vitamin than nothing at all. Better to spend the money you are saving on something healthy, though, rather than on sweets or fatty snacks. You are probably already spending that much on junk food per month, and the vitamins will last a lot longer and do a lot more for you.

Take the multi, and try supplementing with other vitamins, such as the C, and B vitamins if you feel low on energy. Visiting a nutritionist might also be savvy in this case, to evaluate what your system needs and may be lacking. But you really can't go wrong with a daily multi.

A word of caution: remember that moderation is key; be careful not to take any mega doses of beta-carotene, or fat-soluble vitamins, such as E or A. Some recent research has indicated that too much of a good thing could actually have a possible adverse affect on mortality.

As they say, everything in moderation.

CHAPTER 11: SUGAR AND AGING

Here's another reason to cut back on the candy. If your sweet tooth is still overriding your brain's logic center: some recent research has shown that sugar may be linked to premature aging of the skin. Fat or thin, this could affect your face your skin tone, your looks[27]. In essence, that candy that costs $0.99 cents may seem like a cheap treat, but it isn't compared to an $89 night cream, a $200 facial treatment, a $2000 acid peel to soften wrinkles, or ultimately, a $10,000 facelift. People generally guess that I am about six or so years younger than I am, and I attribute it to two factors: wearing sunscreen daily since age 17, and avoiding pure sugars as much as possible.

And beyond the vanity of wrinkles, there are more serious potential issues to worry about. Various studies presented by the American Diabetes Association have linked white sugar, as well as high glycemic-index starchy carbs like white bread, to an inflammatory response linked with a number of dire diseases, including diabetes, cancer and heart disease.[28]

This stuff scared me. Now, I am not just a lover of cakes and cookies. I am a reformed hard-core candy addict. Swedish fish, jellybeans, sour patch kids, gummy creatures, I used to crave it all intensely: now, now so much. I think about what it does on the inside, the artificial colors and flavors and how I'm pumping my system full of chemicals, and it is truly frightening.

Because, of course, we literally are what we eat.

And, artificial sweeteners may seem like a handy way to have your cake and eat it too. But, a study by the journal Behavioral Neuroscience ("A Role for Sweet Taste: Caloric Predictive Relations in Energy Regulation by Rats") has indicated that they can actually wreak havoc on insulin levels and create cravings, perhaps just as harmfully as sugar can.

I found sugarless gum, and protein bars of the lower-carb variety sweetened with artificial sweeteners, to be a major help to me early on, especially lower carb and calorie, vitamin-packed protein bars. But some of the side effects of eating them too frequently had me cut back as I was losing the last 10 pounds in particular. Because once I had a piece of sugarless gum, I wanted a second, and a third, which can lead to something the artificial sweetener people term "gastric distress," which I will say without further elaborating on the subject. It is pretty self-explanatory. If not, let me just say that it involves frequent trips to the latrine (i.e., toilet).

The same principals of breaking the cycle of quote-on-quote addictive foods, and the philosophy of this book, could be taken into giving up other vices-such as smoking. Decide you really don't want to smoke anymore, admit that is pretty much a solid fact that it is terrible for you. And, it will cost you a fortune in health insurance and possibly long-term health care costs. Needless to say, it will just cost you a fortune in general. What used to be a cheap habit (all right, vice) now costs some $9/pack in New York City. At a pack a day, that's more than $3,000 a year in cigarettes, popularly dubbed "cancer sticks" by society.

After I wrote this, I saw that New York City had picked this up this savings concept as an advertising slogan, in a similar mindset. And think what your medical bills could be. Even if you are lucky enough not to get cancer, you could need oxygen tanks for emphysema, or who knows what, all costing quite a lot.

Buy a car (well, maybe not in New York City) or go to Hawaii on that dream vacation instead. And, just think of how much you might save on possible related future hospital costs, for treatment from emphysema, or worse.

I have seen people that I know don't make as much as me (and as a journalist, that hasn't often been a lot) puffing away outside the building — are they trying to slowly commit suicide because they are despairing that they don't have any money? Maybe they would have cash if they would quit the habit, lessening their depression and desire to smoke. It really is that healthy. And on the subject of banning unhealthy substances, look at the moves that restaurants have made to ban trans fats, due to the devastating effects of hydrogenated fats on the human body http://www.webmd.com/content/Article/71/81217.htm.

And if you think smoking makes you think I can attest, after following the smoke trails of obese New Yorkers waddling down the streets of Manhattan: it does not. Perhaps cruelly, I sometimes want to take a picture of someone overweight smoking and post it online as a cautionary tale. As I write this, a relative, always fit, but a longtime smoker, is ill with Stage 4 lung cancer. The drug should be banned.

CHAPTER 12: INSURANCE AND HEALTH COSTS

Of course, possibly or probably reducing the risk of diabetes, heart disease, cancer and other maladies by cutting down on the unhealthy snacking will help you save money in other ways: on your health and life insurance and health care costs.

It costs more per a year for a non-smoker to receive health insurance in some states – and life insurance. According to a study by Duke University, the cost of smoking per day is about $40 per pack over a lifetime, in a 2004 study, not even factoring in the skyrocketing cost of smokes in places like Manhattan.[29]

Life insurance cost is also important, especially if you get sick from bad habits. The bottom line is that you will likely save thousands of dollars in hospital costs, medications and other health expenses if you simply take charge of your health, and drop the weight that has been linked to heart disease and diabetes, two of the biggest killers.

CHAPTER 13: MOVE IT: GETTING FIT

Beyond reducing the amount of useless, nutrition-less calories you are eating, staying as active as possible will also eliminate the calories about to be stored, or already deposited, as fat. But it is easier said than done.

In this technology driven era, children and adults alike sit, more often than ever. We roll out of bed toward our programmable coffeemakers, drive to work and then grab more coffee from the machine a few steps away from our desks. We even shop online, purchasing with a few clicks versus strolling around town or at the mall, or getting takeout or groceries delivered via the Internet, versus going out and dining or shopping. All this quote-on-quote efficiency translates to hundreds of calories not being burned, per day.

As a reporter, exhausted after pumping out story after story, I used to fantasize about a setup where I could lie in bed while I wrote, with a nice flat-screen monitor on my ceiling. That kind of lifestyle would probably have left me hundreds of pounds overweight and possibly even housebound.

Ironically, sitting and lying around can possibly lead to more of the same, while exercise can actually invigorate you. A study recently showed that moderate exercise, such as brisk walking, can actually reduce — not add to — fatigue[30].

Based on my own experience, I believe it. The last thing I, or any of you, probably want to do is to jump on the treadmill or elliptical trainer after work. But by doing some striding at a moderate pace (in the "fat burning" versus "aerobic" range), you will get to catch up on your TV or magazines, burn calories and gain an energy boost, all at the same time.

Don't say you don't have time for exercise if you watch so much as 20 minutes of TV a night. Buy a cardio machine such as a treadmill, stationary bike or, my favorite, an elliptical trainer, and workout while watching, at night or in the morning. Or, do some exercises with free weights. Or, do some jumping jacks, run in place, and try some sit-ups. There's no excuse! And if you say you're too tired, remember, again, exercise can actually give you a boost, revving up your engine to run more efficiently. When I exercise, I can feel it unleashing energy.

Basically, the bottom line is that we have become too efficient for our own good, efficient meaning able to do many things with little to no physical, calorie-incinerating, effort. What translates to a whole lot of convenience and efficiency has had a disastrous impact on our waistlines.

Who am I? Just a person who's found great success with this program, who wanted to share how she did it. Not wanting to become the next Susan Powter (remember her?), infomercial queen Suzanne Somers or, though we all love him, Richard Simmons (who can forget him!), or to become famous for the sheer fact I dropped the equivalent in fat poundage to that of the weight of a toddler, horrifying as that sounds, I just want to help other people, ideally, do the same thing I fought with: get rid of unwanted fat and live a healthier lifestyle.

CHAPTER 14: REMEMBER DON'T BLAME YOURSELF: SURVIVAL OF THE FATTEST

Now, to lose weight takes determination and self-discipline, but self-hatred is just self-destructive, and in my case, stood in the way of taking charge and changing my life. Rather than sighing with despair in that dressing room mirror, or recoiling in disgust and desperation at the doctor's office when you realize you weigh approximately one entire kindergartener more than you thought you did, try to remain calm.

We are designed to store calories thriftily. It is what kept our ancestors from starving and rather, surviving and thriving in times of famine. However, most of us are typically lucky enough to have enough food on our tables at all times, which in general can lead to overeating. Most of us are just way too good at storing calories as fat.

Studies even show a nasty little hormone, leptin, may be a reason why we get hungrier than a tiger at a petting zoo when we diet.[31] Researchers recently found that leptin has observable effects on brain chemistry, making it really hard to keep that fat off, to make a long story short.

In an odd way, it helped me to accept that there was nothing "wrong" with gaining weight. The body simply prefers to store fat when excess calories are available.

Some cultures even celebrate extra poundage; take a trip to a major museum and that will be clear. Think Rubens paintings of robust, plump or outright pudgy, but beautiful women, or the well-padded hips and fat rolls of fertility icons.

In fact, the truth is that not enough fat stored in a female has the potential to lead to impaired fertility, because it can disrupt the monthly cycle of hormones. This is why some competitive athletes do not menstruate, at least when training and maintaining extremely low body fat percentages[32]. On the other hand, too much fat, can also possibly lead to impaired fertility, because raised insulin levels have been linked to PolyCysticOvarianSyndorme (PCOS).[33] One can still be "thin" in terms of having a low weight on the scale for one's height, but still have a body fat percentage that is in the healthy range.

It's all about finding the middle ground, and the healthy weight for you — not some idealized supermodel weight, or your senior prom scale number — just a weight that will keep you living healthily, as well as possible, for as long a time as possible.

We were meant to spend much of our time hunting and gathering, expending hundreds of calories in the process — not sitting around in front of computers all day, and part of the night. Watching TV, downloading mp3s, sitting around and chit chatting on phones. We are supposed to be out and about.

I definitely have a "caveman" or, I suppose "cave woman" type of metabolism, in the sense that I store fat very easily, often, I suspect, simply by looking at food (well, that would be a bit of an exaggeration). If I were stuck on a barren desert island, or stranded in the Andes after a plane crash, I would definitely be one of the last women standing. Odd as it is that waifish genes should be attractive, defying centuries of Rubenesque body types being the ideal that is the way things go nowadays. Despite the J.Los of the world, there are still plenty of fragile-looking fashion victims out there, who think that skinnier is better, or to use the cliché, that "thin is in."

More seriously, I had struggled with my weight on and off since puberty, when I suddenly started packing on pounds. Various studies over the years have shown the influence of heredity on body weight, and there is definitely a tendency toward weight gain on one side of my family — not morbid obesity, but significant overweight. But it was also a matter of lifestyle, and liking, and eating too much, food.

Still, even morbidly obese people, with not 20 or 30, but 200 pounds to lose, have done it, and slimmed down. And you can, too.

CHAPTER 15: YOU CAN BE TOO THIN

This is apparently a cultural, not a biological, attractor, however. Skinny isn't necessarily sexy — and it might not even be healthy. Being underweight has been linked to a weakened immune system and increased mortality rate, and some studies have even found, shockingly, that having a slighter higher-than-normal BMI — in a range from 25 to around 30, so not obese, but with some extra pounds, has actually been associated with longevity[34].

I felt peer pressure and trimmed down to 120 pounds when I was in high school — again, at 5'9", but realized it was ridiculous to try to be so skinny — and that it just didn't feel, or look, good.

By the way, another reason that it may not be a great idea to get too thin; it may move your BMI into "can't model in Spain" territory — below 18.5. Even the extremely slender supermodel Giselle Bundchen supposedly gained a few pounds to make it over this mark, as reported by CNN.[35]

Another reason is that it may actually make you less attractive. And who wants that? Clothes tend to hang well on women built like coat hangers, but they are modeling the clothes, not themselves. I have been to multiple Fashion Week shows, and the models are all generally 15 or 16 years old, beanpoles having their adolescent growth spurt, rails that hold the cloths like masts hold sails. It is not reality.

Attraction appears to be a very subjective, personalized characteristic, but it seems that for women, for instance, men prefer a BMI around 20.85[36] This is rather slim, but certainly not anorexic.

If this convoluted array of information weren't confusing enough, one major research study actually has indicated that people who are on the more robust end of their healthy weight ranges actually live the longest.[37] Those with a BMI of 25 tended to live the longest, though this study did not account for weight-related diseases, just lifespan.

One recently published study even claims that those who are moderately overweight — not obese, but maybe 10 or 15 pounds over the norm, actually may live relatively longer. The study was extremely comprehensive, a blue chip, gold standard kind of deal.

Yet, some other studies claim it is better to be as low in the healthy BMI range as possible, with a minimum amount of body fat[38].

What is my suggestion, based on my own practice? See what weight and training level you feel best at — the most capable, most energized, most generally healthy, and try and stick with that. What weight don't you get colds at, or feel exhausted at? What weight do you feel strong and fit at, does your body seem to perform best at? Find a weight that is easy to maintain, without a major struggle, within healthy parameters.

So, this diet isn't about getting down to "I can't model in Spain" weight — with a BMI of 18 or less. Unless you are genetically predisposed to be 5' 11' and 105 pounds — typically only possible when a teen is having a growth spurt and shoots up like a beanpole — don't go there. Not everyone is meant to look like Kate Moss, nor would many people want to, with more curvy body types coming back into fashion. Being underweight has been linked to osteoporosis and other maladies[39].

Losing weight should not become an obsession with a particular number on the scale. It is mainly about getting healthy — for your own body.

CHAPTER 16: WHAT TO EAT?

This is up to you-and your own conscience. As mentioned at the beginning of this book, you need to be accountable for what you consume, and take a good look at yourself in the mirror. Spend money on reasonable amounts of healthy food, and do not waste it on fat-filled, nutrition-poor calories.

Is it carbs that seem derail your diet efforts, either because you seem to gain weight from them easily, or because you can't stop eating them? I for one know that if I am alone with a box of cookies or crackers, something bad is about to happen.

If you gain weight from fatty foods like red meat, make sure to eat leaner cuts, like sirloin, and to have them prepared so they're cooked as much as possible, reducing the fat in the meat.

As mentioned earlier on, cravings and binging patterns can vary greatly from person to person — some want sugar, others go for fatty fare. If you do not have a clear sense of what your body runs best on, I recommend that you visit a nutritionist, or even visit an online diet site, such as ediets.com, that tailors plans to individuals' metabolic types and fitness levels.

CHAPTER 17: WHAT TO DRINK: BOTTOMS UP?

Now, here's a topic that isn't often mentioned in diet books as far as I have read: drinking. There is a body of research that indicates that alcohol can cause weight gain due to the affect it has on fat metabolism[40]. It is, at any rate, filled with empty, nutrition-less calories. I drink, but in moderation. Drinking in moderate amounts, such as approximately one drink per day, has actually been said to be the healthiest way to live, according to a study of 40,000 people by the Cancer Research Center in Honolulu (G., et al. Alcohol intake, body weight, and mortality in a multiethnic prospective cohort. Epidemiology, 1998, 9(6), 654-661).

Substances such as alcohol, a substance with molecules that mimic the shape of estrogen, is processed differently in men's and women's bodies.

Alcohol mimics the shape of estrogen molecules in the body, according to research, and may even have an impact on estrogen-sensitive cancers, like some breast cancer[41].

Not all tumors feed on estrogen and estrogen-related molecules — but some do.

And the clear fact is, many alcoholic beverages tend to be full of sugar — hundreds of extra, empty calories.

So, calorie-packed margaritas may taste delicious, and be a great choice once in awhile (preferably, featuring a miniature umbrella garnish and served cold on a warm beach), but, if you are in social settings where have a beverage or two is the norm, there are more calorically efficient ways to get your buzz.

If you like it sweet, have soda water with a splash of cranberry and vodka, or just a flavored vodka and club soda.

As mentioned seemingly bitter, innocuous gin and tonics pack an unwelcome punch (and while mentioning it, stay away from sugar-filled punch, and eggnog. But those should be obvious). And the seemingly harmless diet-cola and rum combo may seem to save calories, but as noted, the sweetener could spark further cravings.

Surprisingly, the right six-packs — of lighter beer — can actually help you maintain your own six pack.

And when in doubt, have a glass of red wine — it is not only low in calories with a relatively high alcohol content, it is apparently filled with powerful antioxidants, giving you a health-conscious reason to say cheers.

Everything in moderation, though: this old adage couldn't be truer, to my way of thinking.

CHAPTER 18: ON DIETS

I am not even a fan of the word "diet." After all, it does contain the word "die," and for those who love eating well, this sort of restrictive existence can be a depressing one, that feels like a living death of sorts. It can certainly zap the fun out of daily life.

Our culture, many cultures, center on eating, as a center of family life, of social gatherings. Think about how few activities we engage in do not involve food in some form.

It sounds so simple to simply eat less, exercise more. To make the calories burned exceed calories consumed. But, in theory at least, this is actually exactly what you need to do to drop a few pounds.

Of course, the body has an amazing ability to maintain its weight. Eat too little, your body will veer into starvation mode and cling to fat, lose muscle mass, and after a temporary weight loss, cause you to gain it all back again rapidly — and then some. And who wants to go through their workday hungry? I certainly cannot.

It is downright depressing how efficient the body is at conserving fat.

Fat is the body's last resort as a fuel source. If you eat too few calories per day in hopes of losing weight, typically under 1200 (see calculation method for approximate calorie needs http://www.bmi-calculator.net/bmr-calculator/), your body can switch into starvation mode, any nutritionist or trainer will tell you. It will cling onto your fat stores, which are energy rich, and burn muscle instead if it thinks you're short on food.

It takes extreme self-discipline to avoid the vending machine as the afternoon slump and daily deadlines hit at once. Levels of hormones produced by the thyroid gland, which controls the metabolism, naturally dip in the late afternoon, leading to many of those 3pm-to-4pm cravings according to nutrition gurus.

Plus, so much of our society is based around eating, eating, eating: brunches, lunches, dinners, drinks: it all ads up to some very unhealthy inches around the midsection.

There are many reasons to want to lose weight: for better health, to look better, because your doctor told you to. Again, there is a mountain of scientific evidence linking excessive weight to diabetes and heart disease, two of today's biggest health problems — and both major killers.

CHAPTER 19: CALORIC RESTRICTION

There is even a school of thought, based on more research available at http://www.calorierestriction.org/, that cutting back on calories can actually prolong our life spans. The theory is that caloric restriction sets off enzymes in the body that push the lifespan beyond the norm. In rats, that is. In people, theoretically, this would translate to a lifespan way outside the norm — somewhere about 120 years, supposedly.

Now, some people may behave like rats, but of course we are not actually rats. A few brave, and hopefully not-too-hungry souls are currently using themselves as Guinea pigs, engaging in caloric restriction to gauge the benefits. They are betting that they will live longer tomorrow, even if they are depriving themselves of eating pleasure, and satiety, today. There are also some researchers who say that the effect of caloric restriction merely returns the rats to their normal state of eating (i.e., not over consuming food). (cite http://sageke.sciencemag.org/cgi/content/abstract/2001/6/pe 3). There are studies being conducted on monkeys as well to gain a better sense of whether or not it holds true for humans.

However, it may take quite a while to see if there's any merit to severely cutting back on food for human beings. The idea of eating like a rabbit to possibly live longer like in rats would work for me, as long as there happened to be enough empirical evidence to back it up. Right now, it's only a theory. I for one don't want to live this kind of monastic existence the rest of my life without knowing pretty much for sure that it will work.

CHAPTER 20: FEELING FULL

One of the most irritating things about cutting back on food is, well, being hungry. Even when the spirit is willing, the flesh can be weak once those hunger pangs set in. They can be incredibly distracting. And with a demanding job, and most jobs require intense concentration and long hours, the waistline often comes after the paycheck in order of importance.

This is a problem that derailed my own weight loss efforts for years. When I was on deadline, I needed to think about the story I was writing — and not have an imaginary cartoon-like "thought bubble" with a pizza, diet cola or chocolate bar in it floating above my head.

What worked for me was eating small meals, regularly. If I restricted what I ate too much during the day, I would overdo it at night. If I let myself get hungry to the point I was starving, I noticed it hampered my weight loss efforts. As mentioned, eating too little will just slow the metabolism down, and your body will cannibalize your muscle mass for the protein before it touches the fat according to slews of research.

Fat is your body's last resort when it comes to fuel. It is an energy-rich calorie storage mechanism in your body, and carbohydrates, and protein, are both burned first when the body doesn't have any food options to choose from in the digestive tract.

CHAPTER 21: EAT FREQUENTLY

I often noticed, working at various "The Office" type corporate campuses, that there was that one employee who stayed as lean as could be, but seemed to eat constantly. There is science that backs that up, that continually fueling your body keeps it burning calories. And some current diets are more about when you should eat that what, many suggested that, to get the body in fat-burning mode, that people consumer five small meals a day, so they are never hungry.

The only problem I have had with eating so frequently is that, though it keeps me from overeating during dinner, it was difficult not to eat too much during a lunch or dinner out, often padding the overall daily calorie count to a level where I was not losing weight.

CHAPTER 22: SEEMING DEPRIVED

Another thing that I, like most people cutting back on calories, cannot stand is the felling of being deprived. When that inner dialogue pops up that says "EAT CHOCOLATE NOW," there really isn't much else that's easy to concentrate on, you know what I mean?

There are many diets that apparently do this, but I found on my own that it was easy to swap some gut-inducing food favorites with some more benign, even healthy versions.

For instance, ice cream. Chocolate ice cream, with chunks of chocolate and gooey, caramel-type stuff in it. There is no way I would want to permanently eradicate the substance from my life. But in the midst of losing weight, its high caloric toll, and price tag (be it soft serve or Häagen-Dazs) were both prohibitive.

So, I took some fat-free, protein and calcium packed Greek yogurt (or strained plain yogurt), and added some flavored protein shake powder and pure cocoa powder to it. I even sprinkled in some chocolate chips. And, at a total of 300 calories for an entire package, only about 100 for half the container, I could eat and satisfy both my hunger, and my craving, without blowing my daily calorie count.

Same thing is true with pasta. I am, as my surname might suggest, part Italian, and do enjoy it, but it doesn't love me back. Not to mention, I feel sluggish after eating it. I don't know why spaghetti is touted as a great food for marathon runners: I don't think I could run a block after downing some fettuccini alfredo, or even some linguini marinara, without keeling over. And I don't mean right after eating; I mean hours later. It just fails to energize me.

One of the foods I first tried was a reduced carb, fiber packed (again, filling) soy-based pasta, with more grams of protein and fiber and fewer per serving than traditional pastas. It is actually fairly tasty, extremely filing, and dirt cheap compared to most other protein sources.

Eggs are also an inexpensive and easy way to get some good protein and nutrition into your system. Look at the nutrition information; eating well is just plain common sense, something most of us have in spades.

And all these years, I think that those candy cravings I was having were actually for fruit, which is much lower in calories, and actually possessed nutritional value. Surprise, surprise, it actually even tastes better!

Vegetables are clearly a top choice, though, in terms of price, they can be expensive. They are worth it, but meanwhile, a vegetable juice drink like V-8, or a low-fat, low-sodium vegetable soup, like gazpacho can provide a good stand in, and I like to keep it on hand. A quick swig can help reduce cravings, and adds some nutrient packed veggie servings to the day. Low-fat cottage cheese and some tomato juice are a great, filling snack or light meal.

Just read the labels! Even if a restaurant does not post the nutritional information on the wall, it will probably be online, as well as calories counts for many basic foods.

FIBER

Palentologists studying our early ancestors found that humans could tolerate up to 100 grams of fiber a day — today we are lucky if we can manage to eat 20 grams daily, quite a reduction[42]. Fiber promotes feelings of fullness, and if our ancestors started out eating huge amounts of fiber, it might explain why we don't feel full when we don't. But other studies claim that we didn't each much fiber at all[43].

Whichever was the case, fiber, or bulk, fills the stomach and digestive system and tricks the mind into thinking that you're full of things that are a lot more calorie-rich than they are. A sugar cookie may have zero grams of fiber, so it does not feel like you are full.

To mimic this effect, try eating more fiber — fresh vegetables, whole grain, fiber filled cereals, oatmeal. You can then have your carbs — and eat them, too, without fear of repercussions on the waistline like from refined carbohydrates.

Foods with water can also help your body feel full and satisfied. Try one like black bean soup, packed with fiber and protein but with a very low overall calorie count. You will be full for hours, not thinking of how little you can eat, and it will help cut your calorie consumption overall. From personal experience, I have also found that drinking carbonated beverages with food fills me up more quickly, in particular, calorie-free, caffeine-free seltzer.

Eating foods with a lot of bulk allow you to eat more, and not feel hungry or, in my case, moody, an unfortunate ill effect of cutting calories on occasion. For instance, an entire container of spinach — nice and bulky and filling — is 40 calories, while a third of a typical chocolate bar is 200-300. Sure, the salad is, well, salad, but it will fill you up. Check out that entire box of fresh spinach in the produce aisle — it's a big box or bag that's less than 100 calories.

CHAPTER 23: DIET TYPES

As said, I did not go on an actual diet to lose weight. Sure I had tried a couple of them in the past — lost seven pounds on Atkins that I'd gained back, lost weight back in high school eating low-fat food. I also used to constantly have colds and sinus problems in high school. Both too much, and too little dietary fat can have adverse health effects (see http://www.healthcalculators.org/calculators/fat.asp for one handy calculator).

In general the FDA recommendation is that no more than 30 percent of the daily calories in one's diet come from fat — so depending on how many calories you can eat based on your frame size, height, weight, gender (men typically have more lean, metabolically-active muscle mass making it relatively easier to burn calories) and activity level,

THE PREMISE BEHIND A FEW THAT SEEM TO HAVE MERIT:

THE GLYCEMIC INDEX DIET This diet is supposed to put you on a slow burn — like putting a log rather than some crumpled up newspaper onto a fire. If you eat foods with a low glycemic index, like brown rice, they burn off more slowly and steadily than refined foods with a high glycemic index, like white rice. You are putting yourself on a slow and steady supply of energy. I have found that eating this way, versus cutting out carbs altogether, keeps me a heck of a lot more full, and sane.

ATKINS I had actually tried this diet a few years ago, and rapidly lost some weight, (then caught a cold a week later) but it was not easy. The first week is pretty darn strict in terms of the amount of carbs you can eat (fewer than 20 grams from carbohydrates a day). It works, but is tough.

SOUTH BEACH DIET evoking, at least to me, scenes of deeply tanned women (and men) in thong bikinis, this diet is supposed to give you a svelte, beach-ready body with a lower-carb diet. It is less restrictive than Atkins, and encourages acolytes to eat lean proteins such as fish and low-fat dairy products. The antithesis, I always think, of the 'beached whale diet,' the eating methodology is what most people have adopted.

There are tons of other diets out there to explore, if you decide you need a more structured plan to go along with

my plan: Sugar Busters, etc. and the classic Weight
Watchers. There are also cleanses, but any medical doctor
will tell you that it is scientifically impossible to lose "real"
weight in a week greater than 3 or 4 pounds, max. Those
diets may work well for you, or not, but if you prefer a
more rigid plan, you can follow one of those diets, while
keeping track of the extraneous spending on food.

But again, if you just follow the plan that set forth, you will
lose weight. I could never diet; because I get hungry, so
just keeping it simple worked for me. And remember, no
matter how much weight a diet promises to help you lose
quickly, most experts agree that it is not only practically
impossible to cut out enough calories per week (3,500 per
pound of fat) to lose more than about two pounds weekly,
but that losing more weight than that, because it is likely
due to calorie cutting that causes your body to lose muscle
mass, is considered unhealthy by most nutritionists and
health professionals. Especially when starting a healthy
diet, eliminating salty fast food, you may lose five or so
pounds the first week, due to a loss of retained water
weight, but this is not all real fat loss. Remember — you
are looking to lose fat, not just pounds.

CHAPTER 24: HOW TO COOK

Being thin has become the representation of wealth that being heavy once was. In "olden times," when people had to farm, reap and then prepare and make the food they ate, only the very rich could even afford to be fat. Having some extra girth, like King Henry VIII, was a sign that you had quite the bank account, and a boatload of servants to prevent any possible manual labor that could trim you down, too.

Now, being thin often symbolizes money (how often have we heard the cliché "you can't be too rich or too thin?) It hints at bikini wearing on yachts, advanced skiing in Aspen, and personal trainers, expensive gyms, and custom diets from chefs and nutritionists. Or, having been able to afford some lipo. It's more expensive to eat a healthy diet, in many cases, than to buy a few packages of mac and cheese, bags of cookies, or pints of ice cream. Buying lean protein, low-fat dairy products, and fresh fruits and vegetables definitely costs more.

Depending on your weight and activity level, you need to eat anywhere from 40 to 100 grams of protein a day — and often, getting the protein we need involves eating lots of fat and carbs from around it. Take a burrito — there is some protein in it — meat, beans cheese, but a staggering portion of carbs (a tortilla) wrapped around more carbs (rice). It is hard to find healthy, low-carb takeout.

The way to get around this problem is to prepare fresh food, whenever possible.

"I don't have time" you say. Nobody seems to have time for anything. Or do we? Wasn't technology supposed to make us more, not less, efficient? In that hour you might have spent browsing the Internet for MP3s you could have easily cooked enough food for a week, storing it in that modern day miracle, GladWare. Buy some low-fat tomato sauce, whole grain pasta, broccoli and chicken, freeze up six or seven servings, and you're set. It's easy, and it's inexpensive.

When I have time to cook, I find it relaxing — at least, when I'm not trying to impress family members or guests. And preparing food on an everyday basis doesn't have to be brain surgery, or take forever. By keeping certain staples around, I am guaranteed a hot or cold meal when I get home, eating as fast or faster than I would be if I had ordered takeout or stopped in at the supermarket (and, as my mother has always advised me, never shop when you're hungry).

I have found this especially handy when I was single and living alone, because I either disliked making a huge amount of food or cooking a single meal just for myself, but would get sick of leftovers. The flip side is that I would overeat, because I would make double or triple portions of a particular dish, and be tempted to finish everything off in one session, to avoid the trouble of reheating it later on.

Sure, you can chuck the GladWare when you're done. But think about how much you're saving the environment — from paper and plastic garbage created from the packaging of other foods, if you take the time to rinse and reuse. You'll save money, too. You're not paying for the marketing or merchandising of the food.

Cooking also burns calories: perhaps not as many as cross country skiing or a weight training session, but more than the minimal effort required to punch numbers into the microwave.

The question often hits me; why are we fat? When it comes to food preparation, it all points to one major reason: it is just way too easy to eat. As noted, even rats have been shown to pack it on when exposed to a wide variety of foods to choose from—like our fridges. If only we would just eat when we were hungry — and eat foods that did not create unnatural cravings by driving our blood sugar up and down.

This is when I came up with the concept of this plan, the Charity Diet. Because, facing facts, without some kind of moderate caloric reduction and focus on health, we would just keep on eating.

As noted, the best part about this plan, aside from losing weight if you follow it as described, is that you will save money, and cooking is a great way to both control what you eat, high-quality ingredients, and how much of it you consume. To make 5 frozen meals, your weekday lunches, the cost is about $5-$7 per meal, depending on the ingredients. Even with meat. Divide that into four servings, that's little over a dollar a meal. Compare this to at minimum, the cost of fast food or frozen meals: at least $3 to $5 per day, per meal resulting in a minimum weekly cost of $15 — and this is just the baseline. Multiply this by 52 weeks in the year, $780, versus 260 or 156. You could easily save $500 to $1000 a year, or much more than that, eat well, and then do what you want with the money. Make your own charity — a vacation where you finally pig out to your heart's content, maybe on roast pig at a Hawaiian luau (in Hawaii).

Control — this diet is different, because it's about taking control of your lifestyle. It's not for the morbidly obese, or people who are in serious health trouble with weight-related problems. It's for people who've packed on a few pounds, and need to shave it off.

CHAPTER 25: FOODS TO EAT – AND AVOID

There are a lot of scientists out there, with a lot of theories. The calories-burned-must-exceed-calories-eaten formula is tried and true science, but there are some additional opinions.

On carb sensitivity: As said earlier in this book there are those that can seemingly simply glance sideways at a bagel and gain a few pounds. There are theories of insulin resistance, which makes it harder to burn fat. There is no one diet to suit everyone's metabolism, and there are simply biological hints you must follow in order to eat what's going to make your system perform best.

There are supposed "good foods."

Scientific research has found that there are some pretty surefire foods and phytochemicals to eat that are winners, based on some of the following compounds:

There is a book about "Power Foods" that features research on a variety of powerful substances, phytochemicals, thought to help the body. Lycopene, found in tomatoes,

Polyphenols, Reservitrol, found in red wine; these are just a few of the "wonder compounds that scientists are beginning to analyze and understand.

Of course, this is based on recent research that could be turned on its ear in a year or so. After all, how many years was it that the scientific community believed that the Earth was flat, before Galileo, considered a heretic, said it was actually round? There is solid research showing that these chemicals have some health benefits — but season that conventional wisdom with a grain of salt.

Generally, foods like vegetables and fruit are filled with these types of healthy compounds.

But at minimum, aside from a varied diet centered on healthy foods, such as veggies, take your vitamins. At the very least, take a daily multivitamin, and some supplemental water-soluble vitamins, since you will be drinking a lot of H20 that will flush them out of your system, such as Vitamin C. The Nobel Prize winning scientist Linus Pauling was a major advocate of Vitamin C and improved immunity, and it is vital to your skin's collagen production, important as you slowly but surely lose weight and want to maintain good skin tone.

THE BAD ONES: FOODS TO AVOID

Aside from the obvious sugar- and fat- filled items, avoid trans fats in particular: New York City actually BANNED these fats, as if they were an illegal substance on par with crack or heroin. The effect they are alleged to have on the arteries is, well, disastrous. They are very similar to hydrogenated fats, fats that basically have a hydrogen molecule attached to every available place, and, to the point we care about, cause disastrous effects to the arteries.

INSULIN, HUNGER AND THE GLYCEMIC INDEX

At first, I believed that the key for me was eating low-carb foods. But sometimes I would feel off, or a total lack of energy after consuming such a meal. I realized that it was not just the low carb, but low glycemic index foods that were a trick toward shedding fat. Such as oatmeal, high-fiber cereal, low-carb pasta, and so forth. These are stick-to-your-ribs carbs that burn off over hours, and keep you feeling satisfied, and energized.

CHAPTER 26: EXERCISE TYPES

Exercise is still a relatively new thing for us (meaning, humanity) — starting in the 50s and 60s and expanding in the 70s, as running came into vogue, and the 80s, when aerobics became popular. There are more exercise fads than I can, or would want to count, here.

Our ancestors had it tough — growing their own food, hunting their own dinners, building and repairing their own homes.

CARDIO

I used to think that cardiovascular exercise was a joke. I come from a family where running was generally seen as something one does to get away from something, not a recreational or fitness activity. And running seems to burn only a ridiculously miniscule amount of calories per hour, despite what seems like tremendous effort. I would always wonder after that painful first ¼ mile — can the calorie count be RIGHT on this darn thing? However, I found that there were some major benefits once I started hitting the "hamster wheel ("you know, the treadmill…)

I have been doing cardio for years, and did not lose much weight without following the charity plan as well. But it did two things that were key.

One, it suppressed my out-of-control appetite. When I was just lifting weights, I would get so incredibly hungry afterward that I would consume more calories than I had burned. Cardio helps burn the fat off, especially first thing in the morning, experts say, since your body is already in fat burning mode after sleeping, before breakfast.

Two, it was a matter of doing the right kind of cardio. Running, good, but I was no track star back in high school — I had a note that excused me from running the mile in gym class due to asthma. In fact, I never ran a mile until my late 20s. And while I enjoy it, it can be painful. The key is finding something you like. And for sheer efficiency, I prefer the elliptical trainer. Jump on that for 30 or 40 minutes 4 or 5 times a week, and the pounds will melt off.

I am not, and never plan to be a marathon runner myself. The potential side effects — chafed skin, lost toenails, are not worth it to me, nor is the tremendous investment of time put into training. And, some marathon runners I have known have developed related health problems including a hip replacement in one runner's 30s, and chronic pain conversely proportional to how many marathons the person had run. The blood blisters I developed from running on an incline on the treadmill were disgusting and painful enough — and that was from running only two miles — not 20.

To me, unless you are a gifted runner with a chance to set some records, or excel in another grueling sport, the point of exercise is this: Keep your body functioning at its best and able to do all of the things you want to do, without overdoing it to the point of obsession or injury. Do what feels good, for you; what you like to do, what seems to make you, personally, fitter; not what "seems" to be right. And if all else fails — just walk, if you can, as much as you can. Take the stairs (but, not if they're in a creepy apartment stairwell, of course); try and make each moment of the day an opportunity to make your body fitter.

It may seem like a lot of time — but think about how many hours you spend sitting on your couch watching television. You could watch the same shows and get fit simultaneously. Or read a magazine — or whatever. It's not so bad, exercise!

WEIGHT LIFTING

I will admit that this area still confuses the heck out of me — but I am not alone in this. In general, it is believed that by building and maintaining muscle mass, our bodies perform more efficiently, and burn more calories even when we're just sitting around watching "American Idol" afterward.

I am not a fitness expert by any means. Try circuit training under the advice of a certified personal trainer if you can afford it. I didn't want to make that investment, and frankly did not like the few free sessions I had with a personal trainer (paying someone to boss me around? Not my idea of a good time!)

The bottom line with resistance training (using an exercise band, or gym machine) or weights — be they lighter weights or heavier, is that you are strengthening your body and priming it to burn fat more rapidly and efficiently. You need to put stress on your skeleton to strengthen your bones, and one of the only ways to do that effectively is to lift weights, to force the bones to repair themselves and take in more calcium.

YOGA

I have mixed feelings about yoga. As someone who repeatedly failed the "sit and reach" test in high school, where one bends forward over the legs to test flexibility (I'm sure my ultra muscular hamstrings were to blame), doing moves such as the "downward dog" can be rather uncomfortable — even painful when I was overweight. I took classes for awhile, but must have had an unhappy expression on my face after one particularly boring session, where half the time was spent in downward dog, and the instructor, no waif or fitness icon herself, who was directing, but not actually performing, any of the yoga moves, asked "do you like doing yoga?' and my answer was no.

But I have since had a change of heart. I think that there is probably a form of yoga for everyone. It can be relaxing, and really get you limber. And there is always one particular svanasana, my favorite pose (the corpse pose, lying flat on one's back with the arms by one's side, often covered with a highly comfy blanket). I also like Pilates quite a bit, which focuses on core strength of the abdominal muscles, and was originally developed by Joseph Pilates to help injured dancers recover and get back in shape.

CHAPTER 27: ENVIRONMENTAL IMPACT

In cutting back on snacks, sodas, fancy coffee drinks and pre-packaged meals, you will also trim the girth of garbage piles. Think about how much junk you produce each day, often by eating what your body considers trash anyhow.

I saw "An Inconvenient Truth" three times, after having already started this book, and based on the research in this documentary and elsewhere, there seems to be little question that global warming is a reality.

Every time you get takeout, think about the cardboard, plastic, and paper that you're using once then throwing away.

Feel good, knowing that you are producing less plastic, paper and cardboard waste that creates pollution being destroyed or even recycled.

And speaking of the environment, there is also the dire possibility of a global food crisis at hand[44], due to massive temperature changes, as well as demand for food that is outpacing supply. Temperature-related droughts and heat waves are killing off crops, and even affecting the way nature has adapted; for example, producing a hospitable climate where honeybees can thrive, and then pollinate the crops properly. No bees means no healthy fruit trees[45]. It is a lot of doom and gloom, but seems pretty well justified.

However, there are estimates that eating healthier foods and returning to traditional farming could cut energy consumption in the U.S. food system by 50 percent.[46]

We also might want to focus on needing fewer calories per person to get through the day, because there might be fewer calories around to consume.

SAVE SOME FOR SOMEONE ELSE:
FOOD MAY OR MAY NOT BE RUNNING OUT

There are some other, more dire reasons to cut back on consumption. If what scientists claim about global warming is true, we may have a major food shortage on our hands in the next few years that will affect vegans and carnivores alike.[47]

Global temperature changes may lead to declines in crops. There might not be enough fresh water to irrigate land. Vital farmland could flood globally.

And even something as seemingly small as those little bees could mess everything up. Due to mysterious factors, possibly cell phones, or perhaps illness, bees have been getting lost on the way back to their hives, and dying. They are not doing the job that they evolved for millions of year to do — to perform the role of cross-pollinating plants and crops through their flowers, to both fertilized the plans, and ensure that there is a healthy genetic mix among the plants. Despite all of the scientific advance in agriculture, losing the amazingly efficient assistance of the bees in keeping farms going could have a disastrous impact on crops, impacting everyone, not just the vegetarians, since the cows and chickens need grass, too.

And based on supply and demand, and a very real possible shortfall of food, at least relative to the bountiful crops we've been used to, the price of food is skyrocketing. This is making what we eat – rather, what we don't eat — even more important to our bottom lines.[48]

There is no question that Americans live in one of the greatest societies that has ever existed. Now "greatest" refers as much to our collective waistline as our other accomplishments.

But there is one 800-pound gorilla, so to speak threatening to stomp all over our success: We are exceptionally overweight.

Hopefully my book sheds some light on the big question, why the heck did we get so fat?

There are some very simple reasons that we have gone from thin to, well, thick.

Food is overly accessible: food is an industry

People are programmed to crave variety.

We sit on our rears all day: we are built to roam for hours in search of food, to hunt or till fields until there is no tomorrow. First with television, then with the microwave. We expect modern health care to come up with magic bullets to cure everything that ails us, rather than work to prevent diseases, like heart disease and type 2 diabetes, that are not necessarily inevitable.

After seeing your 20th infomercial on fitness in a tube, abdominal contraptions that make Fisher Price toys look like sophisticated scientific instruments and diet plans guaranteed to melt 40 pounds of flab away results not typical — with moist eyed sycophants praising the plans to high heaven, you might be ready for a change. I was, despite the cheap or not-so-cheap thrill of being able to melt that fat away in a heartbeat.

The plans also struck me as playing into the excess that created our bloated society to begin with. Paying more money, for more stuff, to eat or do in addition to all the other things we consume and spend time doing — it just seemed too much. For some, exercise and diets have become the religion of the last few decades, worshiping not fatted calves, but anorectic racehorses as icons. Designers cut the dresses for size two runway models, and are then worn by size zero actresses on the red carpet. Anyone who doesn't fit this ideal is called out and ridiculed by the tabloid press. The idea of spending my money on some kind of diet program was vaguely sickening.

There is just so much excess junk in our lives — and in our trunks.

We have been brought up to consume, whether it's clothing, cars, or food. Adopting this plan is a way to take control of your consumption — of how much you eat, and what you spend your hard-earned dollars on.

CHAPTER 28: THE HAPPY BEGINNING

You don't really need to eat that. Just remember this, because there are so many opportunities to overeat.

If you are hungry, by all means, eat. But just be careful of what, and how much, you consume. You don't really need to eat a cheese Danish when a protein bar would do. Test yourself with this method: keep a healthy snack, I like low fat string cheese! Balance bars, in your desk at work, so when the 4pm munchies roll around, you have a good option available. If you have a taste craving for mini-choco donuts, but don't want the snack that's on hand you're not really hungry. Find healthy substitutes for the foods you crave — like fresh raspberries instead of gummy bears; they're a lot more satisfying. And a lot healthier — worth the price, and still money saving since you'll probably go buy something else to eat after the sugar shock from the candy wears off (in more scientific terms, the insulin crashes).

By using this book to approach food and fitness in a practical, efficient way, you will hopefully gain the same reward I did: weight loss, and better overall health. It is not a fad diet, but a lifestyle change, that helps you keep track of what you are spending to feed yourself — and how you can make a change.

CHAPTER 29: KEEPING TRACK

What are you doing with your savings? How much weight have you lost? Write me at mediacy@gmail.com.

This is a lifestyle, and as said, a philosophy, and see how you, and everyone else, is making a positive difference in their own, and others' lives.

A percentage of the proceeds of this book will be donated to charity

Lose weight, save money — help both bottom lines.

CHAPTER 30: FOOD DIARY/DAILY PLANNER

DAILY PLANNER (SAMPLE): **ESTIMATED CALORIES AND MONEY SAVED PER DAY**

BREAKFAST:
ESTIMATED MONEY SAVED (EMS):
ESTIMATED CALORIES SAVED (ECS):

LUNCH:
EMS:
ECS:

SNACK:
EMS:
ECS:

DINNER:
EMS:
ECS:

TOTAL DAILY SAVINGS:
TDEMS:
TDECS:

EPILOGUE:

This book can help you lose weight and save money at the same time, with virtually no effort. Developing and following this plan helped the author lose excess pounds and pay off all of her debt in the process. Her weight loss method is simple to follow, based on time-tested health information, and takes up virtually no time during the day, making it easy for even the busiest people to stick to. It is less a diet than a lifestyle philosophy, by a busy Manhattan-based editor who had packed on some pounds and racked up some credit card bills and found the solution to both problems. It will change the way you think about calories, educate you on some of the latest news on weight loss, and convince you that now is the time to take control of your health and finances. It can be used alone, or in conjunction with other diet plans, but if you are not the type to weigh out each chicken breast you eat, or obsessively track each calorie you consume, this is the book for you.

ENDNOTES:

---

[1] See U.S. food pyramid information:
http://fnic.nal.usda.gov/nal_display/index.php?info_center=4&tax_level=2&tax_subject=256&topic_id=1348)
[2] See CDC info, and related article at
http://www.medicalnewstoday.com/articles/42134.php
[3] U.S. Department of Health and Human Services National

Institutes of Health (NIH):

http://www.nhlbi.nih.gov/new/press/05-10-03.htm

[4] Centers for Disease Control and Prevention (CDC)
http://www.cdc.gov/nchs/fastats/overwt.htm
[5] From Journal of Animal Science, Society of Animal Science: http://jas.fass.org/cgi/reprint/74/10/2355.pdf

158

[6] See *Yale Scientific*: article, "From 'Supertaster' to the Taste-blind':
http://research.yale.edu/ysm/article.jsp?articleID=77

[7] From seattle pi: cited from the NY Times, specific article not cited:
http://seattlepi.nwsource.com/health/289113_healthrail19.html

[8] Reuters article dated August 26, 2008: "Monkeys Experience Joy of Giving Too, Study Finds":
http://www.reuters.com/article/scienceNews/idUSN2525835320080826

[9] From SeniorJournal.com: Jan. 23, 2008 article by Christe Bruderlin-Nelson, Contributing Writer, Health Behavior News Service
http://seniorjournal.com/NEWS/Eldercare/2008/8-01-23-FewStrategiesExist.htm

[10] Number of anecdotal citations online and research studies, NPD Group research; also see "Fashion's Invisible Woman" article on http://articles.latimes.com/2009/mar/01/image/ig-size1

[11] See my article from *DSN Retailing Today* magazine, July 21, 2003, "Casual Male enters heavyweight advertising: George Foreman to bring golden touch to big & tall apparel":
http://findarticles.com/p/articles/mi_m0FNP/is_14_42/ai_105988948/

[12] Article, ScienceDaily.com, Aug. 20, 2008: "Obesity Raises Risks Of Serious Digestive Health Concerns: Incidence Of GERD, Colorectal Cancer Increase With Body Mass"
http://www.sciencedaily.com/releases/2008/08/080819160237.htm

[13] See article The New York Times, June 13, 2008, "Japan, Seeking Trimmer Citizens, Decides to Measure Millions of Waistlines":
http://www.nytimes.com/2008/06/13/world/asia/13iht-13fat.13680954.html

[14] Article from American Public Health Association, "California Bans School Junk Food," http://www.apha.org/membergroups/newsletters/sectionne wsletters/oral/fall05/1988.htm

[15] *Psychology Today* article, April 5, 2009, by John Cline, "Sleep and Teenagers", "Sleepless In America" http://www.psychologytoday.com/blog/sleepless-in-america/200904/sleep-and-teenagers

[16] From *Obesity* (2007) 15, 253–261; doi:10.1038/oby.2007.512, "Short Sleep Duration is Associated with Reduced Leptin Levels and Increased Adiposity: Results from the Québec Family Study" http://www.nature.com/oby/journal/v15/n1/full/oby200751 2a.html

[17] American Heart Association, Heart Disease and Stroke Statistics — 2009 Update: http://www.americanheart.org/presenter.jhtml?identifier=303 7327

[18] CDC Foundation, Diabetes: Are You At Risk? http://www.cdcfoundation.org/healththreats/diabetes.aspx

[19] See glycemic index information, http://web.mit.edu/athletics/sportsmedicine/wcrglycemicind ex.html

[20] American Diabetes Association, *Diabetes Care*, "The Prevention or Delay of Type 2 Diabetes" http://care.diabetesjournals.org/cgi/content/full/25/4/742?m axtoshow=&HITS=10&hits=10&RESULTFORMAT=&titl eabstract=delay&searchid=1017670620764_65&stored_sea rch=&FIRSTINDEX=0&fdate=4/1/2002&journalcode=dia care

[21] See Health Bulletin, "Caffeine Prevents Parkinson's — and More" http://www.healthbulletin.org/herbs/herbs5.htm

[22] Duke University, DukeHealth.com, "Cutting Caffeine May Help Control Diabetes" http://www.dukehealth.org/HealthLibrary/News/10226

160

[23] *The Journal Of Nutrition*, "Quinides of Roasted Coffee Enhance Insulin Action In Conscious Rats — Shearer et al" http://jn.nutrition.org/cgi/content/full/133/11/3529/F1

[24] University of Maryland Medical Center, Green Tea http://www.umm.edu/altmed/articles/green-tea-000255.htm

[25] MedHeadlines.com, "U.S. Life Expectancy Shorter for Many" April 22, 2008, citing Harvard School of Public Health and University of Washington findings http://medheadlines.com/2008/04/22/us-life-expectancy-shorter-for-many/

[26] WebMD.com, July 8, 2008, by Miranda Hitti, "Keeping Food Diary Helps Lose Weight" citing August 2008 edition of the *American Journal of Preventative Medicine*

[27] Multiple research studies, including citation at ScienceDaily.com, "Not So Sweet: Over-Consumption Of Sugar Linked To Aging"

[28] Senior Magazine Online, "Sugar and Aging, Sugar's effect on the aging process" http://www.seniormag.com/caregiverresources/articles/sugareffects.htm

[29] *The New England Journal of Medicine*, "The Price of Smoking" http://content.nejm.org/cgi/content/extract/352/20/2143

[30] ScienceDaily.com, Mar. 2, 2008, "Low-Intensity Exercise Reduces Fatigue Symptoms By 65 Percent, Study Finds" http://www.sciencedaily.com/releases/2008/02/080228112008.htm

[31] Studies: Leptin reverses weight loss–induced changes in regional neural activity responses to visual food stimuli; J. Clin. Invest. Michael Rosenbaum, et al. 118:2583 doi:10.1172/JCI35055

Also, Revisiting leptin's role in obesity and weight loss; J. Clin. Invest. Rexford S. Ahima, et al. doi:10.1172/JCI36284).

[32] The Journal of Clinical Endocrinology & Metabolism, "Amenorrhea in Female Athletes Is Associated with Endothelial Dysfunction and Unfavorable Lipid Profile" http://jcem.endojournals.org/cgi/content/full/90/3/1354
[33] WebMD.com, "Clomiphene Best for PCOS Infertility" http://www.webmd.com/infertility-and-reproduction/news/20070207/clomiphene-best-for-pcos-infertility
[34] *The New York Times*, "Causes of Death Are Linked to a Person's Weight" http://www.nytimes.com/2007/11/07/health/07fat.html?_r=1&ref=health&oref=slogin
[35] CNN.com, "Skinny Models Banned From Catwalk" http://www.cnn.com/2006/WORLD/europe/09/13/spain.models/index.html
[36] Research, University College London and Newcastle University, cited in "Score The Perfect Figure" http://www.dailymail.co.uk/health/article-353625/Score-perfect-figure.html
[37] BBC News, "Overweight People May Live Longer" http://news.bbc.co.uk/1/hi/health/4468001.stm

[38] Fred Hutchinson Cancer Research Center, "The Breast Benefits From Low Body Mass and Exercise" http://www.fhcrc.org/about/pubs/center_news/2006/oct19/art1.html
[39] The American Journal of Clinical Nutrition, "Putting Body Weight And Osteoporosis Into Perspective" http://www.ajcn.org/cgi/content/abstract/63/3/433S
[40] From thefactsabout fitness.com, "Why Alcohol Calories Are More Important Than You Think" http://www.thefactsaboutfitness.com/research/alcohol.htm
[41] Physorg.com, "New Animal Study May Explain Why Alcohol Consumption Increases Breast Cancer Risk" http://www.physorg.com/news97034599.html
[42] NCBI, Pubmed.gov, "The Ancestral Human Diet: What Was It and Should It Be a Paradigm For Contemporary

---

Nutrition?"
http://www.ncbi.nlm.nih.gov/pubmed/16441938
[43] Medanth.org, "Applying Medical Anthropology: Gut Morphology, Cultural Eating Habits, Digestive Failure, and Ill Health" By John A. Rush
http://www.medanth.org/case_studies/rush01.htm
[44] Global Policy Forum, Mar. 3, 2008, Katarina Wahlberg, World Economy & Development in Brief, "Are We Approching a Global Food Crisis?"
http://www.globalpolicy.org/socecon/hunger/general/2008/0303foodcrisis.htm
[45] Ecovote.org, "Bees: Another Global Issue That Should Not Be Overlooked" http://www.ecovote.org/blog/?p=69
[46] ScienceDaily.com, "Eating Less Meat And Junk Food Could Cut Fossil Energy Fuel Use Almost In Half"
http://www.sciencedaily.com/releases/2008/07/080723094838.htm
[47] Reuters, By Brian Love, May 29, 2008, "Food Prices To Stay High As Biofuels Blamed"
[48] Reuters, By Charles Abbott, May 19, 2008, "U.S. Food Price Rise To Be Largest In 18 Years: USDA"